HUMAN SEXUALITY IN NURSI

best wishes

Jean Glover

Human Sexuality in Nursing Care

JEAN GLOVER, SRN, RCNT, Dip. in Human Sexuality
(London University)

Nursing Officer, Family Planning and Psychosexual Counsellor for Peterborough
Health Authority.
Tutor to the Course for the Diploma in Human Sexuality, St George's Hospital
Medical School, London.

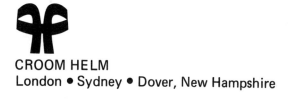

CROOM HELM
London • Sydney • Dover, New Hampshire

© 1985 Jean Glover
Croom Helm Ltd, Provident House, Burrell Row,
Beckenham, Kent BR3 1AT
Croom Helm Australia Pty Ltd, First Floor,
139 King Street, Sydney, NSW 2001, Australia

British Library Cataloguing in Publication Data
Glover, Jean
    Human sexuality in nursing care.
    1. Sexual disorders——Nursing   2. Sick
    ——Sexual behaviour
    I. Title
    612.6'0024613   RT87.S49

ISBN 0-7099-1141-6 (pbk)

Croom Helm, 51 Washington Street,
Dover, New Hampshire 03820, USA

Library of Congress Cataloging in Publication Data
Glover, Jean.
    Human sexuality in nursing care.

    Bibliography: p. 153
    Includes index.
    1. Sick – Sexual behavior. 2. Nurse and patients.
3. Nursing. 4. Sex (Psychology) 5. Sex (Biology)
I. Title. [DNLM: 1. Counseling – nurses' instruction.
2. Psychosexual Development – nurses' instruction.
3. Sex Behavior – nurses' instruction. 4. Sex Disorders –
nurses' instruction. HQ 21 G565H]
RT87.S49G57 1984   612'.6'0024613   84-19881
ISBN 0-7099-1141-6 (pbk)

Printed and bound in Great Britian

CONTENTS

Part V Referral 145

FIGURES AND TABLES

Figures

Table

To Bill, my tutor, who gave me the freedom to write.

PREFACE

I was delighted to be asked to write this book as I feel there is a gap between books written at some length for the sex therapist or psychosexual counsellor, and books written for the layman about male and female sexual functioning. This book has been written with the nurse in mind and stresses that the sexual part of a person is an integral part of that person, and, as such, will need to be taken into account when dealing with *all* patients. The book also stresses the important, constructive role that all nurses can play in the identification and early management of sexual problems as they present in patients.

It is written for post basic students in fields such as stoma care, psychiatry, midwifery, health visiting, family planning and gynae-cological nursing to name but a few. The book would also give an overview of the subject to nurses attending the Joint Board of Clinical Nursing Studies Course 985 – 'The Principles of Psycho-sexual Counselling'. However, it throws light for all nurses, includ-ing student nurses and those in Baccalaureate programmes, on one particular facet of all people – some of whom may become their patients.

Throughout, I have used the word 'nurse' to include midwives and health visitors and referred to them as 'she'. This includes male nurses. Patients are referred to as 'he' unless this is inappropriate. The word 'patient' has been used in situations where 'client' might seem more appropriate, particularly in the United States of America, but 'client' has been reserved for formal counselling situations when he will be seen by a 'counsellor'.

ACKNOWLEDGEMENTS

I should like to thank those who made it possible for this book to be written – all those involved in my training as a marriage guidance counsellor; Dr D.M. Cockin, who initially trained me in sexual counselling in the family planning clinic; my Director of Nursing Services, Mrs P.J. Williams, who has always encouraged me to develop my speciality; my colleagues at St George's Hospital Human Sexuality Unit for consolidating my ideas; the patients from whom I have learned so much over the years and from whose experiences I have drawn.

Thanks are due to typists, Margaret Aldridge, Linda Aschettino and Dulcie Mitchell; Deniss Ingall for drawing figures 5 and 6; Ann Cowper who gave permission to reproduce figures 10.1 to 10.4 from her *Family Planning* (Croom Helm, 1981).

A special thank you must go to Jane Selby, friend and colleague in family planning, for her constructive criticism throughout the writing of the book; to another friend (who wishes to remain anonymous) who told me when I was writing nonsense; to Ann Cowper for reading the final draft and to Gill Lurie for her help in compiling the index.

I have greatly enjoyed writing the book, and thank my family, and the many friends and colleagues who have helped and supported me, for making it possible.

INTRODUCTION: THE SEXUALITY OF THE PATIENT AND THE ROLE OF THE NURSE

People, including nurses and patients, have many needs, some of which, such as the need to breathe, eat, sleep and eliminate, are basic to survival. They have needs for warmth and shelter, and each individual has his own needs for work, achievement and self-esteem, for social contact and sexual contact. Each of us has a unique personality, and sexuality is an integral part of that personality.

When a person becomes incapacitated by illness, he becomes labelled a patient. Because he is unable to see to all his needs for himself, the nurse's role is to be concerned with those needs until such time as the patient can care fully for himself. Traditionally, the nurse's role was to feed, wash and dress the patient, to assist as necessary with his bladder and bowel functions, observe his *medical* condition, report changes to the doctor and to carry out the treatment for that condition as prescribed by the doctor. As the nurse's role became more specialised and mechanically complex, increasing emphasis was placed on treating the condition rather than the patient.

More recently there has been a swing towards viewing the patient as a whole person, with an increasing understanding by the nurse that treating the medical condition is only part of the answer, and that there may be other factors integral to the patient's well being.

In viewing the patient as a whole, there seems to have been a tendency to ignore the sexual side. Regardless of whether or not the patient says anything about that aspect, it is there. It may be that being ill affects only his ability to have sexual intercourse with his partner – both because he is in hospital and because he does not feel much like it. But it may be that his medical treatment directly affects his sexual functioning – examples such as drugs for hypertension producing impotence or a stoma affecting his body image. Outside hospital it may be that small children are making the mother too tired, or that she has a poor self image as a woman and therefore no longer feels sexual. It may be that the contraceptive pill is depressing her libido.

The sexuality of the patient is important to him, but it is often ignored. This may be either because the nurse (and possibly her

1

teachers) is too ignorant or embarrassed to consider those needs, or because the patient is too embarrassed to ask the questions that he needs answering. These together lead to a conspiracy of silence.

The nurse may run away from the problem, feeling that the doctor is the appropriate person to deal with the sexual aspect of a patient's medical or surgical condition. Indeed, in many cases, she is right that it needs a doctor to decide whether or not there is some particular physical or psychological problem.

But sexuality is not just about sexual intercourse or even just about relationships between people. It is also about our concept of ourselves as men and women – about our manliness or femininity as we see ourselves or as we would like to be – about our appearance and behaviour and the effects we hope they will have in attracting those who matter to us. It is about the fears and fantasies about ourselves and others. The patient may need to share these fears; need to feel that someone will listen uncritically and without embarrassment; need someone to help him and to explain why he feels as he does. The nurse is there at hand. Whether she likes it or not she is the only one to fill this need.

It does not call for medical knowledge but just a little imagination to realise for instance that a man who has a mid-thigh amputation of both legs might be worried that he will have difficulty with intercourse if he has only ever done it in the traditional missionary position – the man on top of the woman. Or there is the very common situation where the woman has had an episiotomy during childbirth. Nursing and medical staff rarely mention anything about how the woman might feel when intercourse is resumed. She may well fear that she will experience some pain. She may even fear that she will split open again but, at the same time, be reluctant to mention these fears.

The fact that often no one says anything to patients about the sexual side of themselves reinforces in them the suspicion that it is not 'nice' or 'normal' to have sexual feelings and needs or appropriate to mention them. If all is not well sexually when they return home from hospital they may feel that there is something wrong with them, and with no one to talk to, may think that no one else feels as they do.

The sexual aspect of patients is not just about their concerns with sexual performance – that is the narrow view of sexuality. What also concerns patients is their body image in cases of scarring after extensive burns or after mastectomy or colostomy operations.

Patients may experience fears such as 'How could anyone want to look at me, never mind having sex with me – having only one breast, or a smelly hold in my middle?' – 'Will I ever be touched again?'.

What the nurse can do is not necessarily to *treat* sexual problems, as this needs specialist training which the nurse may undertake alongside other disciplines such as social workers, psychologists, doctors and marriage guidance counsellors. But probably more important is that the nurse who has an open and accepting manner and an understanding of the sexual aspect of the patient and, therefore, feels competent to deal with the situation, can help to *prevent* sexual problems developing.

The health visitor or public health nurse is ideally situated to help her patients who may not have any medical problems and, therefore, will not be seeing any other health worker. She, while visiting the family, can listen for that half-hidden comment or question that patients use to introduce something that they are shy or reluctant to talk about. She can, within her total care of her patients, deal with queries regarding the patients' sexuality – or indeed that of their children or parents.

Midwives are another group who work with women who are at a particularly vulnerable time of their lives. During pregnancy and in the puerperium the woman's body image changes and her body is subject to dramatic hormonal changes, and trauma of some degree occurs to her sexual areas. An understanding and sensitive midwife may prevent the onset of sexual problems.

The school nurse is in a position to be in touch with teenagers in schools at the time of their lives when their sexuality is developing. She could assume the role of the significant adult which is a necessary part of a teenager's development.

Family planning nurses are especially concerned with the sexual side of women, dealing as they do with women of child-bearing age. There are approximately 35 years in a woman's life when her need for contraception may bring her into contact with family planning nurses more often than any other nurse. Women, and men too, often choose family planning nurses to reveal their sexual anxieties to. This may be because many nurses selected for family planning training have the sort of manner and attitudes that will encourage patients to reveal their anxieties, and part of the training reinforces their interviewing skills and their ability to deal with patients' sexuality.

Even staff of a children's ward need to be aware of the strains that continual visiting will put on the sexual life of the parents. The nurses must also be aware of the emerging sexuality of children in their care; particularly of long-stay, mentally or physically handicapped children who will not develop and go on to have adequate sexual relationships if they are deprived of the sex education that is a necessary part of everyday life. This group is particularly neglected as far as an understanding and acknowledgement of its sexual needs is concerned.

The sexual needs of psychiatric patients and adult mentally handicapped people often prove to be an embarrassment to staff. There appears to be a conspiracy of silence amongst staff dealing with these patients so that, particularly in long-stay psychiatric hospitals, furtive sex in the bushes, for example, is condoned as long as staff are not made officially aware of what is happening. Patients who might request a room to be made available in order to have privacy and comfort for a sexual relationship with another patient, would receive, I suspect, very little sympathetic consideration.

I have tried to show that an understanding of patients' sexual needs is part of the role of all nurses, both in hospital and in the community.

It will have become apparent by now, I hope, that when talking about sexual needs I am not just talking about a person's need to have intercourse. What I am trying to introduce is the concept of the person as a sexual being with his appearance, hormones and what are called the secondary sex characteristics – hair distribution, breasts, external genitals and voice – playing a part together with the interpersonal relationships that seem to be an essential part of human life. Sexual needs are very bound up with the emotional needs of love, closeness and caring.

To be able to deal competently and confidently with human sexuality in nursing care, the nurse must have an understanding of how a person develops into a sexual being, an understanding of normal sexuality, some idea of the likely causes of sexual problems and how and when to refer if the problem is beyond her competence. However, the most important requirement is that she must be able to communicate with her patients before she can be of any help at all.

Consequently, I have divided the book into five parts. Part I deals with communication between the nurse and the patient, and looks at some of the requirements and processes of counselling. Part II covers the emotional and sexual development of the individual into a young adult. Part III is about adult sexuality, describing the sexual anatomy and physiology and how sexuality is affected by the person's lifestyle and situational factors. Part IV defines sexual problems and suggests in broad outline how they may develop. Part V concludes with assessment for referral, types of therapy and referral agencies available.

PART I

COMMUNICATION AND COUNSELLING

The interaction between the nurse and the patient is often perceived by the patient as unsatisfactory. It is kept on a detached level by the nurse who seems to be mainly concerned with the clinical tasks that have to be carried out. The patient is expected, by and large, to suffer these in silence.

The patient may have need to talk to the nurse on a more personal, meaningful level, but soon learns either by the response of the nurse or by copying the behaviour of other patients that meaningful interaction is often missing in a nurse/patient relationship.

The nurse may also have needs to relate in a more personal way to the patient. Indeed Hockey (1976) says that one of the common reasons given for wanting to nurse is to have contact with people. However, the nurse soon learns from observing more senior nurses that talking to patients is often not encouraged. The nurse is made to feel guilty for spending time in an apparently unproductive way at the patient's side and may be warned about the danger of becoming 'too involved'. While this danger may be very real, it is not insurmountable given support, but the nurse's response to the warning may well be to shut herself off from patient/nurse interaction in the future.

An opportunity exists for the interaction to become more satisfying for the patient and for the nurse as well if she will allow it, in the history-taking in family planning and in other disciplines such as psychiatric nursing, midwifery and health visiting. Compiling the records for the nursing process also offers an ideal opportunity. However, the nursing process needs to be carried out in the spirit it was intended – to obtain a picture of the total needs of the patient and to plan and implement care based on those needs. Filling in forms is not what the nursing process is about. Until and unless the nurse has a commitment to see beyond the stated 'medical' diagnosis, the chance of the patient's psychosexual needs being recognised is very small. If the nurse is prepared to consider this aspect, then it is necessary for her to have certain skills in communication, an understanding of the counselling role and, perhaps most important, an understanding of herself.

8   *Communication and Counselling*

This first section is an introduction to these subjects and it is stressed, as it is in all sections, that it is only an introduction. There are many books for further reading on the subject and a list of some of them appears at the end of each section. However, communication and counselling are practical skills which cannot wholly be taught in theory, but which must be practised, preferably under supervision, with feedback both from supervisors and from a peer group.

1 VERBAL COMMUNICATION

Verbal communication is that which is spoken and heard in the interaction between two or more people. There are various factors that may influence the perception of verbal communication; some of these are to do with the unspoken messages that are sent at the time – that is, non-verbal communication.

Language. An ability to speak the same language would usually be seen as a prerequisite for verbal communication, although much can be conveyed by tone or gesture.

However, speaking the same language does not ensure communication of meaning, as, for example, Americans speak English but they may have very different ways of expressing themselves from the British. For example, in Britain a 'rubber' is purchased from a stationer's and is used to 'rub-out' pencil marks. However, in the States, a 'rubber' is a condom or sheath and to 'rub-out' means to kill or to get rid of someone. The American equivalent of rubber is 'eraser' and to rub-out is to 'erase'.

Regional Differences. Even within countries regional differences may mean that the same words will have different meanings. In Britain the northern use of the word 'while' meaning 'until' instead of the dictionary definition of 'during the time that' caused great confusion at railway crossings. The notice 'wait while the lights are flashing' had to be changed as it appeared to have the opposite meaning to northerners.

Accents. These may be difficult to understand but they may also influence the listener in such a way that assumptions are made about the character of the person speaking. This is part of the common habit of stereotyping people, and it is a barrier to accurate perception. Accent may also indicate social class which in turn may have an affect on the listener who may be prejudiced against that class of people.

Jargon. Each job and profession tends to have its own vocabulary. Some words are specific to certain situations whereas other words have become generalised. The word 'paranoid' has a specific psychiatric definition, but it is used by people generally to describe someone who is unreasonably feeling attacked. Nurses may use 'in' words, partly from habit but also as a means of distancing themselves from the patient and emphasising their authority and superiority.

Understanding. Even if two people speak the same language, in a manner recognisable to each other, using simple words, there is still opportunity for misinterpretation.

In family planning, for example the question 'What method of contraception are you using now?' may elicit the response 'None'. The unwary may write down just that. The more experienced nurse will realise that it can mean 'I am not having intercourse', 'We are using no method of contraception', 'My partner is using a sheath or withdrawal' – in other words I am not using a method of contraception.

Expression. The inability to express oneself is the opposite to misunderstanding the answer. Several people involved with communication as part of their job have this notice on their wall:

> I know you *believe* you understand what you *think* I said, but I am not sure you realise that what you *heard* is *not* what *I meant*. (Jack Dusty, 1981)

This sums up the difficulties of verbal communication. If the person who is trying to talk cannot accurately put into words what he is feeling, then what chance has the listener of getting the message right?

The nurse who speaks with and listens to the patient needs to understand how all these factors will affect both her and the patient's perception of what is being said.

2   NON-VERBAL COMMUNICATION

This is the name given to those messages which pass between two or more people in many other ways apart from speech. These messages may be deliberate as in the case of teenagers who dress in a certain manner to show each other and the world outside that they belong to a particular group. Another example is the sober-suited businessman who wishes to be seen as conforming. Nurses use the non-verbal communication of their uniform to pass on the message that they belong to the organisation and are in charge. Uniform also gives protection to the nurse and patient by indicating that the necessary close body contact is not a sexual advance. It gives nurses to some extent a group rather than an individual identity. This leads to their being stereotyped as nurses rather than seen as individual people.

On the other hand, the person sending the non-verbal messages may be completely unaware that they are being sent and therefore they may conflict with the verbal messages. Someone who fidgets and twists his hands may belie his confident manner of speaking. However, a great deal of literature has been written about the interpretation of the language of non-verbal signals, much of it taken, I feel, to extremes–the way someone rubs his nose for example being interpreted by a whole sentence.

Nevertheless, the ability to understand non-verbal signals plays an important part in assessing the complete message that is being conveyed, particularly if one set seems to contradict the other. There are five main areas of non-verbal communication.

Appearance. First appearances have been shown to be very important in one person's perception of another (Anderson, 1974). We may judge (or think we can) nationality, class, age, sex, occupation, financial status, and as a nurse may try to judge the person's state of health at the same time. Our appearance is often adapted to what seems to be appropriate for the occasion and to bolster confidence. It is noticeable that of patients attending family planning clinics that many of those who are expecting a vaginal examination not only put on clean underwear, but also their 'best' top clothing and some make themselves up very attractively too.

11

In hospital the social sitation is not one of adults meeting in similar clothes but one of patients in night attire and nurses in uniform. This forced change of appearance will affect the inter-action between the two and may result in feelings of dependancy in the patient who is suffering from a sense of loss of identity.

Facial Expression. Of all the facial features the eyes are most used to judge messages (Argyle, 1972). People become disconcerted if they cannot see the person to whom they are speaking. Indeed, if other facial expressions such as smiling are contradicted by un-smiling eyes, then the message from the eyes is the one more likely to be believed. Patients may reply 'Fine' when asked how they are but their eyes may well belie them. Eyes may give other messages such as pupil dilation which suggests attraction. However, it may be a good idea to check that the dilation is not caused by drugs!

Generally, in experiments, people have been shown to be good at judging a person's mood from his facial expression (Ekman, 1971). Nevertheless, cultural differences must always be allowed for.

Voice. This is often a clue to the patient's mood and may indicate anger, depression, happiness, indifference or dependancy. The way something is said may well contradict the verbal message. 'I am *not* angry' said between clenched teeth, with rigid facial muscles and in a loud voice may well lead the listener to judge that the speaker *is* angry.

Volume is often deceptive as some people may speak quietly in a very dominating manner and others shout their heads off most ineffectually. The change of volume is probably more significant than the person's usual volume of speech, although most people will recognise the stereotype of the school ma'am who speaks loudly and orders everyone about (like nurses?) and the meek little hen-pecked man who never raises his voice above a whisper. They are really less common than imagined, I think.

Body Posture and Movement. The way a patient enters a room may say a great deal about how he is feeling; although, particularly with men, bravado must be allowed for. Patients may sit in bed or in a chair with slumped shoulders suggesting dejection or may be up-right and alert suggesting well being. However, it could be that the latter patient is wearing a surgical corset!

Patients undergoing gynaecological examinations and who are

very anxious adopt a common posture of legs crossed and arms crossed over the body when on an examination couch. Anxious male patients have been observed to adopt an identical pose.

As for the nurse, her body posture will give messages to the patient. Standing hands on hips with one foot in the door to listen for the telephone may well emphasise the dominance of the nurse over the patient lying in bed and the relative importance she puts on talking to him. However, if the nurse takes a chair and sits next to the patient, so that their eyes are level, showing that she wants to talk on equal terms, then the interaction may well be very different.

The nurse who is drooping and obviously tired may evince sympathy from the patient and, therefore, induce something nearer equality in the interaction. However, it is probably likely to reverse the roles with the patient feeling that he cannot burden the nurse with his worries as she is too fragile to bear them.

Body Space and Touching. This is an aspect of non-verbal communication that is very dependant on culture. The British on the whole stand further away from each other than in other cultures and have many taboos about touch (Argyle, 1972). For individuals the use of body space and in particular touching is very bound up with their upbringing. Non-touching families produce children who grow up into non-touching adults. One of the common problems in sexual development is lack of touching. People who have been deprived in this way often find it difficult to relate to others in a warm sexual manner.

An understanding of the difficulties of touching and of adequate body space is important to the nurse as her job requires her to invade the patient's privacy and areas of the body are touched which in normal society would not be acceptable. Nurses deal with this by having a detached manner, treating the patient as if he were an object rather than a person; or by being authoritarian and treating the patient as if he were a child because socially it is more acceptable to touch and give personal care to a child; or by laughing and joking to hide both the nurse's and patient's embarrassment and thus denying the situation.

There is no easy answer, but whatever manner is arrived at should include an understanding of the difficulties, of how the patient is likely to be feeling and how the nurse is feeling. An attempt should be made to make the patient feel that he is being cared for and touched in a compassionate way as a person rather than that he is being invaded.

On the whole, people stand nearer to one another the closer they feel and further away if they feel remote or unfriendly (Argyle, 1972). However, for patients the choice of space is strictly limited. They may be confined to bed or to a chair in a small room or have to sit in rows with others. This limitation of their choice of space will affect the interaction. The nurse may use body space to emphasise her detachment by standing at the end of the bed to talk to the patient.

One phenomenon often seen is that of 'the hand on the door'. It occurs in a situation following a conversation when either the nurse is about to leave the patient or, more commonly, the patient is about to leave the nurse. During the conversation seemingly trivial or straightforward things may have been said but as the patient is leaving, feeling safe with his hand on the door as an escape and knowing that further time is limited, the patient says, 'Oh, by the way' or 'I just wanted to ask' or 'I thought of something the other day'. This is likely to be the most significant thing he has said during the interview and will be important to him. It is often something that he wants to run away from, and part of him hopes the nurse will not hear it or that he can get away before the nurse can respond. If the nurse is feeling less than at her best it is easy to miss. It should always be watched out for.

The problem is how to handle it. If the interview is part of a series where the patient can confidently expect to return then it might be appropriate to leave it until the next time as long as it is noted down. However, the safest thing is to pick it up at least briefly by showing the patient that you have heard and will listen. It may be necessary to demonstrate this by inviting the patient to sit down again with you.

An understanding of the use of body space is important in structuring interviews and in arranging meetings of different kinds. The way desks and chairs are arranged in an interview room may indicate what sort of interview it is going to be. The traditional position of the interviewer in a large chair behind a desk with the patient being given a small hard chair on the other side of the desk very clearly tells the patient just what his position is expected to be; whereas two equal chairs on the same side of the desk will suggest to the patient that someone is interested to talk to him. As well as position and relative size of chairs, relative height is important. Try to have a conversation with someone, side by side, with one of you in a high upright chair and the other in a low easy chair.

Interaction in groups is affected by the way chairs are arranged. Chairs in rows with the leader out at the front produces more leader-individual interaction than group interaction. The latter is facilitated best by chairs in a circle. These differences are best tested out for oneself. Try sitting in a committee meeting or other formal meeting around an oblong table in different positions at different times. It may well be found that the ease with which you attract the chairman's attention depends on where you sit.

If you sit in a circle and your chair is slightly in front of those either side of you, you may feel compelled to move back into line as it feels uncomfortable to have others behind you as you cannot check their reactions. Similarly, if you sit slightly back from the others, quite quickly they will adjust their chairs so that they can see you. An empty chair in a circle of people can be quite a disrupting influence as people tend to imagine things about who might be sitting there.

One final thing should be said about all forms of communication, and that is that one person's communication with another will influence the other person who gives feedback about what he has received and how he feels about it. The first person then adjusts his communication to take account of this. Communication is therefore always a two-way process, which is why the word interaction is perhaps more accurate.

3 COUNSELLING

What is Counselling?

Counselling is a word that is used to mean many things and is often used inappropriately. It is sometimes used to mean 'advice giving'. 'I have counselled her to do such and such' is often heard – which usually means that a particular course of action has been suggested.

There is nothing wrong with advice giving, indeed it may be the most appropriate action to take. There is a joke told against counsellors who may be more used to helping people to find out what they want to do than giving advice. 'Man in street to passer-by, "Can you tell me how to get to the station?" Passer-by, who happens to be a counsellor, "What is it about the station that makes you feel you have to go there?" ' This is an obvious situation where advice or information giving would be the most appropriate response and the counsellor's response is inappropriate.

There are times when the person requesting help needs information to make an informed choice. School counselling and career counselling are two areas in which giving information plays a large part. Nurses may be involved in giving advice or information as part of the health education aspect of their jobs. Health visitors and midwives are two obvious examples but, of course, all nurses include health education as part of their work.

Discussing with a patient the use of lubricating jelly and the likely return of sexual feelings after an episiotomy is advice giving, not counselling. Nevertheless, in doing so the nurse has the opportunity to pick up any underlying sexual anxieties that the patient may have and, at the same time, the nurse signals to the patient that it is acceptable to talk about sex with her, if that is what the patient wants to do.

Counselling, as I am using the term here, means helping the client to explore how he sees the situation and allowing him to arrive at his own decision about his problem in his own way. The British Association for Counselling has produced a definition:

Counselling is a process through which one person helps another by purposeful conversation in an understanding atmosphere. It

16

seeks to establish a helping relationship in which the one counselled can express his thoughts and feelings in such a way as to
clarify his own situation, come to terms with some new experience, see his difficulty, and so face his problem with less anxiety
and tension. Its basic purpose is to assist the individual to make
his own decision from among the choices open to him.

The Counselling Relationship

The interaction between counsellor and client, or between nurse
and patient in a similar situation, is what is known as the counselling
relationship. It is a contract between the counsellor who offers her
expertise and the client who agrees to work at his problem. In some
form of behavioural therapy, a written contract is provided stating
what each shall be responsible for doing. Sometimes when the client
pays it is easier for this contract to be acknowledged and this may
put the client on a more equal footing with the counsellor in that he
is then contributing something of worth – as is the counsellor.

It is more difficult to have this explicit contract between counsellor and client in the informal interaction between nurse and
patient, and yet, in order to avoid misunderstandings, it is important
for the nurse to know within herself just what she is offering to the
patient, and it is her responsibility to make her role clear to the
patient.

Because of these requirements it is difficult to 'counsel' relatives
or friends as it is usually impossible to clarify the counselling role
and to detach sufficiently from the everyday situation that the
counsellor may be involved in. Similarly, there is some conflict in
counselling subordinate staff in that it is impossible to relinquish
totally the part of the management role that is concerned with
disciplinary matters. It may be possible to give advice about career
progression and listen sympathetically to personal problems, but, if
these problems affect how the manager will relate to the staff
member in the future then I believe that the counselling is better
carried out by an independent counsellor.

The Client

The Client Must Want Help

This may seem to be a little obvious but, in fact, many clients are ambivalent about wanting help, because one set of needs may conflict with other needs. For example, the need for a sexual relationship may conflict with the need to be separate and alone. In fulfilling the first, he will be denying the second. Most of the phobias surrounding non-consumation in a woman – that is her inability to allow penetration by the man – can be successfully dealt with. However, if there is also a deep-seated fear of becoming pregnant and a strong wish not to have children, then it may be impossible to achieve the declared objective of wanting penetration without activating the stronger fears about fertility.

Sometimes it is found that the client requesting help has been 'sent' by his partner to be 'sorted out'. At other times one partner actually as well as metaphorically drags his partner along to be seen. Under these circumstances it is difficult for counselling to be effective as the resentment felt by the unwilling partner may sabotage the efforts of the counsellor. The counsellor may be able to bring the resentment out into the open, in which case constructive counselling may be achieved. Another problem is when one partner has a significant relationship with someone other than his partner. If he is not prepared to reveal that relationship then it is unlikely that he will accept help to resolve the situation with his partner. Ultimately, the client must want help.

The Client Must Ask for Help.

It has been found that clients who make their own appointments to see a marriage guidance counsellor are much more likely to keep their appointments. Clients who have been 'sent' by other agencies seem less motivated to attend. The most extreme example of being 'sent' is when counselling is imposed as part of a judicial sentence. The counselling of clients by probation officers is very restricted because the clients are forced to attend. Problems may also arise when couples who are seeking a divorce are 'sent' for counselling by their solicitors.

Patients with sexual problems who see their problem as physical may ask their family doctor/general practitioner to refer them to a gynaecologist. If he 'sends' them to a sexual counsellor, particularly if that counsellor is part of a psychiatric department, then the patient may well arrive very angry and unwilling to look at the problem – if, indeed, he arrives at all.

A patient who presents with a problem, such as a family planning problem, or with child rearing difficulties, should have that taken seriously by the nurse even if the nurse suspects that other problems are the real cause of concern to the patient. If the nurse latches on too quickly to the underlying problem without dealing with the presenting problem, then she risks alienating the patient who may feel that no one will take him seriously. The skill lies in balancing taking the patient literally in his request for advice and recognising and responding to the often unspoken message.

Needs of the Client within the Counselling Relationship

Regardless of the problem with which he presents, each client has the same fundamental needs in the counselling relationship.

To Be Treated as an Individual Person. It is easy to fall into the trap of considering the client as a 'case' or a 'problem'. Many clients present ostensibly with the same problem, but each reacts to that problem in a unique way. Each client, therefore needs to retain his identity and to know that *he* is important to the counsellor.

To Be Heard. The client needs to tell somebody what is troubling him. He needs to hear himself speak out loud what has been going around in his head, possibly for a long time. Only then can he begin to acknowledge for himself what he thinks and feels. He needs to tell his story with the minimum of interruptions, encouraged to go on by the empathetic response of the counsellor.

To Express Feelings. As well as recounting the facts about what is concerning him, the client needs to express the feelings behind the words. If feelings are perceived to be damaging, hurtful or too strong, they are often repressed, rather as if they are pushed into a bottle and the cork jammed in tightly. Unfortunately, the good feelings of joy, love, and sex are also pushed into the bottle, leaving the client feeling depressed, weary, and suffering from lack of sexual drive. It is often necessary to enable the client to recognise and release the bad feelings before good feelings can be experienced and enjoyed.

To Be Accepted. Having stated his problem and expressed his feelings, the client's overriding need is to be accepted as the person he is, 'warts and all'. His fear is that he will be thought bad, peculiar, unacceptable; that he will be found wanting, judged and condemned.

Difficulty may arise when the counsellor finds that something the client has said is contrary to what *she* believes. However, acceptance of a client does not necessarily mean agreement or approval of his point of view – only that she accepts him as he is, together with what *he* believes and feels. He needs also to feel that the acceptance is accompanied by a warm sympathetic manner, rather than that he is being merely tolerated.

To Sort through the Confusion. The client may need help to recognise the extent of his problem – indeed the problem with which he presents may not be what is really concerning him. The counsellor will need to help him clarify what he is really saying. He may then need help to sort out an acceptable line of action. However, it is no help at all to him to be *told* what to do. He must decide on his own, and his decision must be something he can live with.

To Be Able to Trust. Although these clients' needs have been listed separately, in practice they do not follow necessarily this sequence with one stage moving into the next. What happens is that the client says something, measures the counsellor's reaction, builds trust, says some more, begins to feel accepted, reveals something more important or expresses his feelings . . . and so on. The degree to which the client feels he can trust the counsellor depends on her response to him, and usually builds up over a period of time.

Part of the trust is to do with the confidentiality of what he is revealing. He needs to feel that he will not be betrayed and exposed to everyone.

'Special Pearl' Technique

Clients or patients who have an underlying anxiety that they will not receive adequate care and support, may play a game in which they subconsciously provoke a certain response in their carers. A patient may give special information to a nurse 'because only you understand me'. This nurse will then be motivated to care for him particularly well – feeling that she must protect him from the other staff who cannot satisfy his needs as well as she. This makes this nurse feel more important than the others.

This manipulation of carers, all of whom may have received the special information, 'special pearl', is likely to set one agency against another, or produce a competitive, secretive working atmosphere for staff. If this situation arises, it is vital that it is recognised and recorded, so that the client or patient can be helped to discover his real needs.

The Counsellor

The counsellor may be someone in a formal counselling setting who will most likely have received training in counselling, or she may be a nurse who is using counselling skills. Either way, the personality of the counsellor is important. She should have a warm approachable manner. This is something that is very difficult to define, but it is the sort of manner that makes the patient feel 'Now, I could talk to her'.

Listening

The counsellor must be prepared to listen. By this I mean really concentrating not only on the words but on all the non-verbal messages that the patient is giving out. It is very exhausting really listening to someone as it means that the nurse must put away any thoughts about herself. She should have the discipline of being able to switch off all outside stimuli, which is why she needs to have privacy, time and freedom from interruption. Listening is a prerequisite for empathy with the patient.

Motivation

The counsellor must genuinely want to help and be prepared to look at her motivation in putting herself in the counselling role. Most people do things which give them satisfaction and try to avoid doing things which are unpleasant or unsatisfying. The fact that the counsellor is satisfying her own needs by counselling is not necessarily wrong; what is important is that she acknowledges these needs to herself. Needs may include liking the feeling of being needed; the need to take on the role of the mother; the need to relate in a close relationship with someone, which is not being satisfied in the counsellor's private life.

Provided that the counsellor faces herself honestly and acknowledges her motivation, then her needs should not get in the way of the counselling relationship. Needs to dominate, to punish, to live vicariously through the client – being a sort of 'peeping-tom' on the client's life and asking unnecessary questions particularly about the client's sexual habits – these are needs in the counsellor that are not likely to help the client. A counsellor who uses the relationship to force her views on to the client is going against one of the principles of counselling – the right of the client to make his own decisions.

Reactions

The counsellor must also be prepared to look at her own reactions in the counselling situation. This is one of the most useful tools of the trade, but it is a skill that needs much practice. As well as concentrating on what the client is saying and shutting out any external stimuli, she must look at her own feelings. It may be that she will realise that she is becoming angry. Instead of reacting in an angry manner to the client she needs to recognise the anger, ask herself why she is feeling it – is it something in her that is reacting to the client or is it the reaction that the client produces in most people? She needs to modify her instinctive angry reaction and maybe share with the client how she is feeling. A counsellor who feels confident in doing this is often able to enable the counselling relationship to grow and develop to the benefit of the client. Indeed, the fact that she is prepared to show the client in a controlled caring way that she has feelings and reactions will help the client to see the counsellor as a real person and will also help the client to express his own feelings.

Sometimes it is impossible to identify just what is happening in the room. The counsellor may stop and say that she is aware of an undercurrent but cannot identify what it is. The struggling together of the client and counsellor to sort out what is happening between them can be very helpful to the counselling process.

As far as dealing with the sexual side of the patient is concerned, anxieties in the patient will trigger anxieties in the nurse. The sexual side of a person is often full of anxieties and guilts from his upbringing and nurses are no exception to this. Unless the nurse is prepared to face her own anxieties about sex, she is unlikely to be able to help her patients. Denial of these anxieties will only cause the patient to deny them in himself. To help the patient with sexual anxieties, a nurse must be unembarrassed and able to use the words connected with sex easily.

Limitations

The counsellor must also be aware of her own limitations. It may be that the type of help she can offer is not that best suited to the client. It is important to acknowledge this to the client. It might be possible to discuss the problems with another agency or specialist who can give the necessary support for the counsellor to continue, or it may be necessary to refer the client to someone else. Often there is a reluctance on the part of the client to be referred elsewhere. The skill in this situation is in referring the client in such a way that he does not feel rejected nor the counsellor a failure.

Support

It is important that the counsellor has support for herself. Despite being encouraged, as part of her training, to continually look at herself, what she is doing and how she is interacting with her clients, it is all too easy to delude herself and to rationalise her actions. She may say to herself, 'Well of course I am doing that because it is best for the patient', when it may be that what she is doing is because of some need in herself. A supervisor or support group with whom the counsellor discusses her cases is essential for the protection of the client and for the continuing development of the counsellor. It is sometimes unpleasant to have a supervisor or one of the counsellor's peers say, 'Hey, what do you think you are doing!' However, even if strongly defending herself against what they are saying, on reflection the counsellor will often realise that they were right to raise the matter after all. One very useful rule of thumb is that if someone reacts very strongly against something that is being said, then there is a good possibility that there is truth in it. This applies equally to counsellors and clients.

Theories of Counselling

There are several theoretical frameworks that the counsellor may work within and it may be that she will follow one or other fairly closely. Indeed, her training will most likely be in one particular school of thought.

However, many counsellors, once trained, will, in following their own development, look at other theoretical models and may incorporate such features as are felt to be useful. In the end, it is the counsellor as a person who is useful to the client not the theory. The theories are tools to be used. The theories that are perhaps of most use to the nurse are those of Carl Rogers (1965), who developed the theme of the client-centred relationship, with emphasis on the 'here and now' rather than on delving at great length into the client's past. The basic philosophy is that the client has resources in himself for growth and development and that the counsellor's role is to help him mobilise those resources.

The Process of Counselling

The process of counselling suggested here is particularly relevant to formal counselling sessions; however, these skills may be used by the nurse to understand and help patients in other situations, however informal.

Create the Environment

This involves considerations of time and place.

Time. Counselling will need time for the client and counsellor to explore the problem areas together. Often an hour per person is set aside, or what is known as the fifty minute hour. This is to allow the counsellor time to get her breath back, so to speak, and write up her notes before the next client.

However, in the situation of the nurse-patient relationship, counselling skills may be used in settings other than that of formal counselling. Nevertheless, time is still important and it is necessary when the patient says 'May I talk to you for a moment?' to make sure that time is available. This might mean arranging to see the patient later in the day on the ward, or at a home visit, when both nurses and patient have the time. In a clinic setting it might be necessary to check that other colleagues can continue with the clinic while the nurse gives extra time to the patient. If this is not possible then a separate appointment should be made. It is irresponsible on the part of the nurse to indicate to the patient that she is free to talk about the patient's concerns and then have to make excuses to dash away.

Having said all that, I am not suggesting that the nurse gives the patient the message that she is too busy to deal with him. The skill lies in making the patient feel that the nurse is interested in him and really wants to listen, and, at the same time, is making sure that time is available.

It is important also to indicate to the patient how long he has of the nurse's time. The same applies in a more formal setting. People commonly structure their use of time according to that available. A longer session does not always prove more fruitful. Patients who know they have only ten minutes can often use it very constructively; it is only if they do not know how long they have that they may never become settled enough to reveal what it is that they want to talk about.

Even so, the use of the 'hand on the door' is a common occurrence, as is the client who always wants to test out the counsellor to see if she will give him five minutes more.

Place. Privacy is one of the most important aspects of counselling. It is not sufficient to choose a room away from other people, but ideally a room should be chosen that has a solid door and no see-through window to the corridor. The outside window should be protected by blinds or curtains and sound-proofing is another factor to consider. Confidentiality is usually taken to mean the protection of records from other people and refraining from discussing the personal details with others. However, confidentiality should also include not allowing others to overhear consultations.

One point to be raised is that of how to handle the situation where a patient indicates that he has a sexual problem in the presence of someone else – perhaps a student sitting in with the nurse. The nurse may feel that it is inappropriate to discuss the problem with the student present. However, the fact that the patient chose that moment to raise the problem suggests that he felt comfortable with the situation as it was – i.e. a threesome. The nurse may ask the patient if he minds the student being present, but it is more likely that the nurse feels uncomfortable with someone else present than that the patient does. The question of confidentiality should have been raised with the student beforehand.

Another consideration when choosing the place is that of freedom from interruptions. This might mean hanging a 'Do not disturb' sign on the door or arranging with the receptionist not to interrupt with telephone calls. One of the biggest drawbacks to counselling clients in their own homes is that it is not possible to control their telephone, families, or visitors. It is very difficult to concentrate on what a cliunt is saying and feeling if children are running around and interrupting.

In formal counselling meetings outside the home, unless family therapy is involved, children are discouraged. The fact that parents continue to bring their children with them, despite being asked not to, often indicates that they do not really want to look at the problem.

Another advantage of counselling outside the clients' home – particularly in marital or sexual counselling involving both partners – is that it removes the antagonists from the battlefield on to neutral territory. It also affords them an opportunity to do something together, without the children. Indeed, coming together to counselling sessions may well be their only activity together. The journey to and from the session may be an important part of the whole experience.

The arrangement of the room is important. Comfortable chairs are preferable but equal chairs are more important. The desk, if there has to be one, should be pushed against the wall and facilities for smokers provided even if the counsellor is a non-smoker and despite the pleas of health educationalists. Clients need to feel as far as possible at their ease and for many this includes a need to smoke. An interview will not be completely productive if the client has been made to feel uneasy by being denied a smoke he needs.

Define What Is Offered

This may involve explaining the role of the agency in formal counselling. A particular agency may have basic rules for functioning and it is important that the client understands what these are. They may relate to payment, missed appointments, or whether or not the counsellor may be telephoned at home.

It is important that the client knows who is the counsellor. She may be mistaken for the receptionist or, in the case of a nurse, for a doctor or social worker. Clients have preconceptions about the role of all these people and it is helpful to explore these expectations of the client at the beginning.

It is helpful also to check with the client why he thinks he is there. In a clinic setting it may be that he thought he was seeing the chiropodist! Anger at being 'sent' may be revealed at this stage.

Clients need to know how long the session is likely to last. In the case of arranged appointments, children may need to be looked after and in an informal ward situation the patient may worry that he will miss his lunch or that his visitors may have arrived.

The clearer the client is as to what is being offered, the more easily counselling will proceed. However, particularly if attending somewhere new, as well as meeting someone new about a problem that is causing great anxiety, the client is quite likely to mis-hear and misunderstand what is being said. It is not uncommon to find that the ground that the counsellor thought was covered at the beginning is really only clarified after two or three sessions.

Listen

The counsellor should attend closely to verbal and non-verbal signals. She should look as if she is listening – staring vacantly out of the window, even if she is listening, is not very reassuring for the client.

Reassurance

If a client expresses something which is painful for him, this may evoke a corresponding feeling of discomfort in the counsellor. She may feel sorry for the client and rush to reassure him – to tell him that all will be well. However, in doing this she is in fact denying his pain; but by acknowledging his feelings, metaphorically holding his hand while he is expressing his anxieties, the counsellor will make him feel that someone really understands and cares, and will encourage him to continue. Reassurance too early often cuts off any further revelation, as the client may instinctively feel that the matter is too painful for the counsellor, or that she cannot be bothered to spend time with him.

In the daily interaction between nurses and patients, over-reassurance and too early reassurance is very common. However, once the patient has been able to express what he feels, reassurance may then be appropriate. This is particularly the case when the patient requires factual information about his condition.

Limit Questioning

If the counsellor asks questions, then usually she will receive answers. However, the answers may not relate to that with which the client is primarily concerned. If the counsellor is uncertain as to what to say, then the easy way out is to ask another question. It is often not very helpful.

There are two types of question. One is closed-ended questions, to which the answer is either 'Yes' or 'No'. These lead to the questioner frantically searching for something to make the client talk, often resulting in a complicated question, to which the client's response may be simply 'Yes'. Open-ended questions, which force the client to say at least something of what he thinks or feels, are questions beginning with words such as 'How, Why, When, What'. However, if the counsellor is really at an impasse, and knows that the client is having difficulty telling her what is really bothering him and yet has not given her the clues to encourage him to express himself further, then it is helpful for the counsellor to ask, 'What is it about the situation that bothers you most?' The answer to that question will enable her to see what areas she needs to help him to explore, rather than her spending time exploring what she *thinks* may be bothering him.

If the client is able to express what he is feeling without too much difficulty, then questions will only interrupt his flow. It is far better to encourage the client with 'Mmm', 'I see' or a nod of the head.

Reflect

Another way to encourage the client to continue saying what *he* wants to say is to repeat the last few words of what he has just said. 'And so you went to your mother's' or 'And you felt like screaming'. This shows the client that you have been listening, have accepted what has been said and would like to hear more. This encourages the client to develop his thoughts further or to go into deeper feelings about the incident.

Clarify

After the client has had an opportunity to say how he sees his problem, it is often helpful for the counsellor to restate what the client has said: 'It sounds to me as if what you were saying is . . . ' This gives the counsellor the opportunity to check out that she has really heard what the client has said and it gives the client the chance to hear what he has said. Sometimes this can be quite revealing to the client, who may then say, 'Yes, that *is* what I think, I had not quite seen it like that before.'

As well as clarifying what has actually been said, it is sometimes helpful for the counsellor to reveal what feelings she has heard underneath the words. Caution is needed here as a client is not always ready to hear how he feels about something. 'It sounds as if you are really angry about that' may be very helpful and may allow the client to express further his pent-up anger. However, it may lead to a denial – 'Oh no, I am not angry.' It could be, of course, that the counsellor is wrong in her perception, but the episode needs to be noted, perhaps to be raised again at a later stage.

Silence

This is one of the most difficult areas to deal with and requires confidence on the part of the counsellor. The inexperienced counsellor usually jumps in with a question. Silence may be allowing the client, who is temporarily lost in his own world, to cast around that world for a thought or feeling that he has caught a glimpse of but cannot identify. It may be what is known as an 'Ah' experience – a flash of insight as something falls into place – or it may be the client and counsellor sharing a moment of joy or sadness.

Silences can be a powerful counselling tool, but they can, particularly at the beginning of counselling, be an indication of the uneasiness of the client who may need help to express himself. The skill is in realising what the silence means. When in doubt it is a good idea to ask where the client's thoughts have taken him.

Negative Feelings

While sometimes a client will only see the good in a situation and the counsellor may begin to wonder why the client has come to her for help, the commonest situation is the one where the client sees everything as bad. There is a great deal of pressure put upon the counsellor to redress the balance. The counsellor may feel that 'Things cannot be as bad as that'. However, if that feeling is expressed, it has the effect of denying for the client how he is feeling *now*. If the client expresses the situation as all bad, then that is how he perceives it, and unless and until the counsellor accepts that in the client, progress will not be made. The session will either develop into a contest in which the client tries to say how bad he feels and the counsellor tries to reassure him, or the client will give up, agree, go away and not return. Reassurance, whilst it can be very useful if it is about information as to what is normal or common experience, has no place in the early expression of negative feelings.

Once the negative feelings have been expressed and accepted by the counsellor, the client may then begin to voice more positive feelings about the situation, without any prompting from the counsellor. Similarly, in the first instance mentioned, once the counsellor has accepted the client's positive feelings and gained his trust, then his negative feelings may begin to be tentatively expressed.

Conclusion of the Interview

It is important to keep to the time agreed, not only for the benefit of other clients that may be waiting, but also because it demonstrates to the client that the counsellor is businesslike and able to keep within her own boundaries. Frequently clients will test out these boundaries.

It is helpful for the counsellor to summarise what has been said and to define clearly what practical help, if any, can be offered. She may state what steps are to be taken before the next visit as agreed by them both. Further appointments should be made if relevant, and the client given the opportunity to write them down. There is some difference of opinion and practice as to whether one further appointment at a time is agreed, or whether a series of future appointments is booked. There are disadvantages to both methods. The first may lead to confusion in the mind of the client as to how often or over how long a period of time he is to be seen by the counsellor. This could be clarified by 'Let us see how much we have achieved in six sessions from now.' The disadvantage of the second is that if a client fails to keep the first of a series of appointments, then the counsellor will be uncertain as to whether to keep open the remainder, or to slot in other clients.

Note-Taking and Record-keeping

The most important facet of note-keeping is that of confidentiality. Notes that have to be written on a patient's case card that is open for other workers to see should be kept to the minimum. Details that are relevant to the counselling relationship should be kept separate and locked away. They may be identified by a code or number. Notes may be used in discussion at a support group meeting, but names or identifying details are never given.

The degree to which notes are made may vary. It is more usual for fuller notes to be made if the counsellor is in training. Sometimes tape recordings are made, with the client's permission, for use in supervision. However, it is not very helpful to record what happened in the counselling session verbatim from a tape recording. What is helpful is to record not only facts, but feelings revealed in the session. Non-verbalised feelings should be noted and any reactions of the counsellor. It may be helpful to underline points to be raised at the following session. It is usually more helpful to record the feel of an interview rather than what was said.

However, a client may use a phrase that seems to sum up a great deal about himself and that phrase is often worth recording as it may lead to instant recall of the interview at a later date.

Views differ about when to make notes. Some counsellors prefer to make notes during the interview, others immediately afterwards, others the next day. If an interview is mainly about feelings then it may be more productive to make notes as soon as possible after-wards. However, if it is about facts, such as taking a sexual history, it may be helpful to take notes at the time, but stop when the interview progresses into an expression of feelings. Note-taking is very individual and each nurse or counsellor needs to explore for herself the different methods. She should also realise that note-taking during the interview will have varying effects on clients.

Informal Counselling

I have discussed formal counselling sessions in some detail. How-ever, the skills used in formal counselling can be applied by the nurse in the one-off session in the ward or clinic. Indeed, only relatively few nurses will be involved in formal counselling and then only after further training, but most nurses, during their working day or night, meet patients who have a need to be understood and to express themselves. The ability to use counselling skills as part of the day-to-day interaction with the patient is a most important part of a nurse's role.

The process of counselling previously described is relevant to an informal session. For example, a nurse may use only one sentence which reflects or clarifies what the patient has said and yet enables her to establish a rapid rapport – particularly if she is seen to be listening. These are not steps which have clearly defined boundaries – moving on to the next after the previous step is finished; but the session with the patient will move from one stage to another and back again in an easy flow throughout the session.

Perhaps the most controversial step is how much is written down about these informal sessions and how much is told to someone else, for example the nurse in charge or doctor. The nurse must indicate to the patient if she feels it necessary to disclose information told in confidence and should explain to the patient why she thinks it is important. As far as writing is concerned, the question that must be answered is 'How necessary is it for someone else to be aware of what has been said?' – notes being made accordingly.

Nurses often underestimate the value of informal counselling, particularly when listening to patients who present sexual problems. The nurse may feel inadequate to deal with the problem and so be anxious to refer the patient as quickly as possible. However, whether or not the nurse is able to offer constructive suggestions is not as important to him as the fact that she will listen and try to understand him.

Similarly, a nurse may feel that the patient should be speaking to a doctor, rather than to her, and fear that in listening to the patient she may adversely affect any therapy which the patient may receive in the future. This is not so. The nurse should recognise that the patient chose *her* because he felt that he could talk to her and it is to her that he wishes to reveal his difficulties. It may be appropriate for him to talk to the doctor later, but if he is rejected at this stage by the nurse, he may well be unable to talk to *anyone* later.

Suggested Further Reading For Part I

Argyle, Michael, *The Psychology of Interpersonal Behaviour* (Penguin, 1972).
French, Peter, *Social Skills for Nursing Practice* (Croom Helm, 1983).
Munro, Manthei, Small, *Counselling _ A Skills Approach* (Methuen, 1979).
Nurse, Gaynor, *Counselling and the Nurse* (H.M. and M. Publishers Ltd., 1975).
Rogers, Carl, *Client Centred Therapy* (Constable, 1965).

PART II

EMOTIONAL AND SEXUAL DEVELOPMENT IN CHILDHOOD AND ADOLESCENCE

The emotional and sexual development of the individual will be dealt with in this part of the book, and will be followed from conception to adulthood (at about the age of 20 years).

Each person is unique, a product of both his inheritance and his upbringing. Thus the nurse needs to learn how the patient has developed into the person that he is in order to understand how his sexuality affects the nursing care that she will give. Part III will deal with how that person's needs and behaviour in the present will be influenced by the situation in which he finds himself.

Inheritance

In attempting to understand how a person has become as he has, the possiblity of hereditary factors influencing his behaviour should be taken into account.

There are arguments about how much of a person's make-up is as a result of his inherited genes and how much is as a result of his upbringing and environment. There seems to be little controversy about factors such as eye colour or blood group, but there is controversy about how much temperament, or the tendency to react in a certain manner, is inherited from parents. It is extremely difficult to separate the influence of the parents on the child from characteristics that the child may have inherited. However, studies have shown (Thomas, Chess and Birch, 1970) that children do seem to have an inborn tendency in how they cope with the changes and dissatisfactions of early life.

Stages of Development

Different writers have classified the stages of a child's development in different ways according to whether the emphasis has been put on educational stages, as with Piaget, or on sexual and emotional development, as suggested by Freud. Erikson divided the stages of growth of the personality into eight psychosexual stages – from infancy to old age.

In presenting an overview of the subject, I have broadly followed Erikson's division of life stages as described by Lowe (1972) in *The Growth of Personality*.

However, I should stress that a great deal of the material is unproven and is an attempt by writers to explain why people have become the individuals that they appear to be. As a person becomes older, it is possible to ask him how he sees the world, but the further back one goes into childhood and finally into infancy, the more suspect may be the conclusions. They are an adult attempt to interpret the world of the child through adult eyes rather than through the eyes of a child.

The other point to bear in mind is that any division into stages, or ages, is arbitrary; children move from one stage to the next at different times, and different children will show the characteristics of different stages at different ages. The child has needs at each stage of development and provided these needs are satisfied then he will progress to the next stage of development. If these needs are not met, he will progress anyway to the next stage, but some of the later responses may be affected by the lack of earlier fulfilment. There is thought also to be a critical point at which these needs exist, so that lack of fulfilment at the correct time cannot later be reversed or 'made up'.

Another factor of the developmental stages is that of regression. Even if one stage has been successfully passed, if difficulties are encountered in a later stage, then the child may regress or go back to an earlier stage in which he was able to function more satisfactorily. This regression may occur when a child has to face the implications of being supplanted by a new baby and often happens in adults when they become ill. Parents exhibit childish behaviour which may well be reinforced by the dependent relationship often encouraged by the nurse.

4   0–2 YEARS

This is the most difficult age about which to draw any reliable conclusions. The infant is born into a world very different from that in which he has grown and developed for the last nine months, although, during its gestation period the fetus has been influenced by many outside stimuli. Chemicals present or lacking in the diet, the hormones of the mother, smoking and alcohol, may all affect the fetus's physical development (Hawkins, 1983), and it is possible that noise and the emotional state of the mother may affect the fetus emotionally.

After birth, the infant needs to suckle to obtain food to survive and also appears to have a need for warmth, stimulation and the touch of soft material (Harlow, 1959). An infant deprived of these may find his ability to relate to people sexually is impaired.

Because the mouth is the focus of the infant's sensations in the early stages, the first stage is often called the oral stage – as described by Freud. The baby is concerned initially with sucking and later, as teeth emerge, with biting. The infant will also use his mouth to investigate things around him.

In this earliest stage, the infant is dependent on someone else – usually the mother – for the satisfaction of his needs of sucking and being handled. How the adult relates to people later in life will be affected by how well the infant's needs are satisfied. Erikson (1963) described this stage as being essential for trust to develop. The infant who experiences the mother figure in the early months as reliably satisfying his needs will come to know that people can be trusted to satisfy other needs.

This produces a deep sense of security in the child and later in the adult, which provides a basis for sharing, and trusting, others in a sexual relationship. It facilitates a relationship in which adults are able to allow their partners to be separate individuals rather than needing them to be an extension of themselves.

The infant who has his needs satisfied will gradually be able to tolerate separation from the mother figure because the trust that has been built up will allow him to believe that even if his satisfaction has to be delayed a little, then he will be well satisfied soon. This acceptance of a delay in gratification extends into adulthood where a person can tolerate and enjoy the anxieties of the sexual tension before orgasm. But someone who cannot delay gratification becomes more interested in the climax than in the preliminary stages.

Some people who have not achieved this basic security seek oral ways of dealing with anxious feelings in adult life. Compulsive eating provides a feeling of well being that is not connected with the food being eaten. Smoking, it is suggested, satisfies the need for something continually in the mouth.

In adults these unsatisfied needs produce people who, in relationships, may be dependent and clinging, needing the other person to satisfy their infantile needs. As this is unrealistic, the likely outcome is that it will drive the partner further away – thus making the situation worse.

Many adults have what I describe as a feeling of a 'hole in the middle'. This is a feeling of being lost, abandoned, hungry, miserable and insecure. If people have learned to tolerate this as a normal, temporary state of affairs that happens on occasion, then this will not hurt their relationships, but if people seek to fill the hole by excessive demands on another person, by sex, eating, alcohol, by buying new possessions or stealing, then they will make unrealistic demands on their relationships with others and will not find the satisfaction they crave.

The need to be touched seems particularly linked with adequate sexual functioning. Harlow (1973), in his study of monkeys, found that adult sexual functioning was markedly impaired in monkeys who had not had mothers, or warm, soft mother substitutes. He found that the presence of other monkeys could redress the balance somewhat, but the isolated, uncomforted monkeys were unable to mount or be mounted.

Certainly, touching seems to play an important part in human sexuality. Adults who have not experienced touching in childhood seem to associate touch only with sex and in particular with orgasm – the end of sex. Others who have been touched in their childhood tend to see touch as part of caring and affection and an important part of sexual foreplay.

5   2–4 YEARS

Erikson (1963) describes this stage as early childhood and Freud gives it the label of the anal stage. It is the stage where the child begins to control his infantile behaviour, partly to satisfy his own desires and partly to satisfy the wishes of his parents.

He learns to walk – although this starts in infancy with crawling and standing. In walking he can better satisfy his curiosity, even more so if he becomes a climber. This immediately brings the child into conflict with his parents and thus begins the delicate balance of what the child wants against the parents' wishes.

The child also begins to talk, and thus develops a stage of greater interaction with his parents. As well as the child being increasingly able to ask for what he wants, he can also say 'No'. Moreover, he is now beginning to have the ability to act out 'No'. Conflict arises and the child begins to realise that 'No' is an unacceptable word, both to his parents and to himself.

The balance that is achieved between allowing the child some autonomy and yet producing an acceptable degree of conformity will shape how the child reacts in adult life.

A major feature of this stage is bladder and bowel control – hence the name anal stage. If a mother regularly 'pots' a child of eight months or a year old, before the child's nervous system has developed enough to recognise what is happening in his brain, then she may achieve early control and feel very proud of herself. However, what has really been achieved is a reflex action – the feel of the potty on the buttocks producing the stimulus to urinate or defaecate. The real control by the child does not usually begin until at least 18 months and often later. The child must have the ability voluntarily to hold back, to talk or at least make known his needs and, preferably, balance alone on the pot or stand at the lavatory bowl.

The way that the mother and child interact over this piece of learning that is necessary for socialisation, will influence how the child develops into an adult. If the mother encourages the child by showing what is expected, praises when the pot is used, ignores failures and adopts a fairly easy, tension-free attitude, then the child will learn the control for himself in a relaxed way.

It is, of course, necessary to arrange the situation in the child's favour – such as making sure that the pot is available, or the door to the lavatory is open and that the child is not so bundled up in clothing that he could not possibly manage for himself. This attitude to toilet training will give the child the beginning of the feeling of his own autonomy, that he can manage for himself, as well as allowing him to experience the pleasure of his bodily functions.

However, if the toilet training becomes a battle of wills between mother and child, then the only way that the child can gain autonomy will be to delay bowel function for long periods. This may lead to chronic constipation in the child and may produce an adult who shows his anger by withholding and withdrawing in a relationship in such a way that he may say, 'What, me?' and make out the conflict always to be the other partner's fault. His attitude may often provoke the partner into open aggression. A deep-seated reason for premature ejaculation may arise from unsatisfactory development at this stage – where the man frustrates his partner's need for him to keep thrusting, by ejaculating very quickly.

The child who never gains autonomy and yet becomes 'dry' and 'clean' may have decided that the conflict is too great and that he must obey his mother. This produces adults who are neat and tidy – always afraid to make a mess, to play, to risk feeling in case they are wrong. They are usually punctual and become very anxious if others do not observe their rigid control. Rigid behaviour, obsessional behaviour, the need to dominate, to win, to put down others are sometimes the result of anal conflict in adults, who continue from childhood to see the world in terms of perpetual conflict and control. Problems in handling potty training may be a contributory cause for those people who see intercourse as messy, smelly and uncontrolled.

Unfortunately, a parent who has difficulty in accepting his own sexuality is likely to be rigid when dealing with toilet training which may evoke in him memories of mess and feelings of shame. Thus the child may pick up non-verbal cues to do with that part of the body which conflict with his own sensations of pleasure. Holding in and letting go can be pleasurable for the child, as may be producing a stool that has emerged from his body all warm and sticky. The child will learn that what is pleasurable to him is not so to the parent; it may be described as 'dirty' by the parent – which comes to mean 'bad'. He learns that his pleasurable feelings produce anxiety for his mother and thus for him and so he learns to deny these feelings in order to be 'clean' and 'good'.

Similarly, touching the penis or vulval area will be pleasurable – almost certainly discovered when the mother bathed and changed the child's nappy, but if the child actively repeats the pleasurable activity then the anxious parent will soon transmit her anxiety to the child either overtly by removing hands, smacking or putting emphasis on the word 'dirty' or covertly by distracting the child and by expressing dismay in her manner and bearing.

In dealing with people with sexual problems which seem to stem from difficulties in childhood, I often see patients who seem to have had a complete lack of sexuality in their upbringing. An example of this was the patient who said that her mother could not bring herself to use the word 'bitch' when referring to a female dog. Sex in any form was ignored. This attitude seems to be as damaging as being actively discouraged from sexual activity.

Another area of sexuality to do with the anal stage is that of the buttocks. There is some suggestion that a certain amount of sexual pleasure is obtained from being spanked. This argument is used as the rationale for banning this form of punishment at school as it is suggested that the spanking will reinforce the sensations experienced at the anal stage, and will encourage them to be perpetuated into adulthood. There is no doubt that spanking and punishment form a large part of fantasy in sexual life – particularly in men who may well as boys have been spanked more often than girls.

The child who successfully negotiates this phase will have laid the foundation for self-control and autonomy. Those who are continually made to feel a failure, messy or bad will grow up feeling shame about their bodies and doubting their own ability to give and receive pleasure.

Sexual Gender Identity

The sense of knowing that one is a boy or a girl begins during the 2–4 year old stage. There is controversy about the relative influence of inheritance, hormonal factors and culture on masculine or feminine traits.

The chromosomes of males and females differ in that males have the twenty-third pair of chromosomes as XY whereas the females' twenty-third pair are XX. The genetic male or female develops rudimentary gonads at about eight weeks in utero, the chromosomes determining whether they become testes or ovaries. The development of the external genitalia then depends on a secretion of testosterone from the testes during a crucial stage of the fetal development. If this occurs then the external genitalia become that of a boy; if no surge of testosterone occurs then the external genitalia becomes female. It is thus possible for a genetic male to be born apparently a female (Begley *et al.*, 1980).

However, children are rarely born without the apparent sex matching the genetic sex and the external genitals are usually clearly defined. When the parents realise that they have a boy or a girl, they tend to dress the child according to masculine or feminine stereotypes and buy it toys to match those stereotypes. Nevertheless, even when children are dressed in unisex clothing and bought equal amounts of toys for girls and boys, they seem to know what sex they are.

Imitation is a feature of the pre-school child and, by and large, girls will imitate their mothers and boys their fathers. Problems may arise when there is no parent or parent substitute of the same sex, a quite common occurrence these days with the increasing incidence of one-parent families. Children may use parents of their friends who are the same sex as themselves to imitate and in this way affirm their identities. There have not yet been sufficient examples of male/female role reversals to study how this affects their children's gender identity.

In addition to imitation, parents will reinforce feminine attributes such as passivity, dependence and talkativeness in girls and reinforce aggression, self-reliance and reserve in boys. However, there seems to be an increasing acceptance of a wider role for men and women and an understanding that traditional masculine and feminine traits may be seen in either sex. It is to be hoped that in the future children will be freer to develop their inherent tendencies rather than being forced into an unsuitable mould.

Problems with gender identity seem to arise when the wishes of the parent for one particular sex of child is very strong and when faced with a child of the 'wrong' sex seeks to force it into the desired sex. Boys may be dressed as girls, given dolls to play with and may even be given a girl's name. They will continually receive the message that boys are unacceptable. This early rearing pattern may, not surprisingly, cause confusion in puberty or even later in life at some crisis point, and may make them vulnerable to some form of transvestism (Bancroft, 1983).

6   4–7 YEARS

The infant has moved from total dependency on its mother; obtained a degree of control over its movements and bodily functions; widened its personal relationships to include its father and now begins to make relationships with its immediate family.

The focus of the child's sexuality moves from its mouth, to anus and now to its genitals – hence the name given to this stage by Freud, the phallic or infantile genital stage. This is not to suggest that the child's awareness of pleasurable sensations in its genitals begins only now. It is rather that the genital sensations present since birth become more predominant at this stage. The child will frequently touch his genitals – if he is allowed to. Little boys are to be seen holding their penises, almost as if seeking for comfort in a very similar way to thumb sucking. Girls have not such a convenient handle. Indeed, a great deal is written about penis envy with Freud suggesting that girls wish they had such an interesting part of their bodies as boys and may wonder if they had a penis once and had lost it because they were naughty. Watching boys urinate may well provoke this feeling. Whereas boys, Freud suggests may feel afraid when they see girls without a penis and fear that the girls have been naughty and had it cut off. How much these feelings in both sexes affect the development of their sexuality is debatable, but children at play do express such feelings.

Boys and girls quite normally seek to explore each others bodies and, providing they are not discovered by punitive adults, will affirm this physical difference and pleasure in this part of their bodies. Games such as mothers and fathers, babies and doctors and nurses are played – all giving the children an opportunity to explore each other.

Masturbation

This is touching the sensual areas of the body, usually the genitals, to obtain pleasure. It is entirely normal. Masturbation may involve some rhythmic movement such as rubbing parts of the body against other objects, or rocking, as well as the direct touching of the genitals. However, many people deny ever having masturbated. It seems unlikely that they are deliberately lying as they will persist in this view even when trust has been established with the enquirer. What appears to have happened is that verbal or non-verbal messages have been communicated by the parents that masturbation is not nice, is dirty or is harmful. It is sometimes called self-abuse and has been said to cause blindness, deafness, stunted growth and madness. Boys in particular may be threatened with harm to the penis or castration. Little wonder then that children who are small may fear that it is indeed masturbation that has prevented them from growing.

These reactions on the part of parents may be sufficient either to block off any further sexual feelings, so that the child does not remember that he masturbated, or to produce great feelings of guilt in children who continue to masturbate.

Because there are many other interesting things for children to do, masturbation, if allowed, will merely be one activity. However, a child who is lonely, bored or unhappy may find masturbation one of life's few satisfactions, and therefore spend a great deal of time on this activity. The solution is not to stop the masturbation but to find out what it represents for that child. It may, particularly in mentally handicapped children, become a behaviour pattern that seriously affects development. There is perhaps some place for behavioural programmes to limit the amount of time spent in this way.

The Oedipal Situation

Much has been written about this by psychoanalysts and the phrase has become common usage without people realising what it is based on. There is a Greek myth that a king heard a prophesy that his son would kill him. To prevent this he arranged for his son, Oedipus, to be killed. However, Oedipus was saved and brought up by a shepherd – and later killed his father without realising who he was. Also unknowingly he married his mother and had children. When he found out he blinded himself and his mother hanged herself.

The story illustrates the strength of the incest taboo – that is that sex between close members of the same family is forbidden. Other taboos are not common to all cultures but the incest taboo seems to be almost universal.

As part of the child's development, he enters the stage where he becomes romantically attached to the parent of the opposite sex. However, it is taking the similarity a little far to say that every child mirrors the story of Oedipus and continually wishes to have sexual intercourse with his mother or her father. However, boys do frequently say that they are going to marry mummy when they grow up and, in imitation of their fathers, may endeavour to carry out caring tasks for their mothers. A boy may resent his father's presence, particularly if the father is away for some time and then returns to re-establish his position, thus pushing out the little boy.

A similar situation arises with girls who may feel romantically attached to their fathers and who will, therefore, see their mothers as rivals. This situation for boys and girls is very complex and fraught with difficulties. In being a rival of the parent of the same sex there is a risk of alienating that parent. This creates an ambivalence in the child – on the one hand wanting, daring to bid for the parent of the opposite sex, and on the other hand being fearful of the reaction of the other parent. This situation seems to create greater conflict for a girl as her primary attachment is to her mother. So that wanting to need and love her mother conflicts with her wish to usurp her mother's place with her father. A boy's primary relationship with his mother is not threatened in the same way when he seeks to replace his father.

Parents who are happy and secure in their own relationship will handle this situation in such a way that gradually the child realises that what is desired is not possible. He will achieve this without too much of his initiative being stifled or being overwhelmed by guilt feelings. He will not have had to compromise his own sexuality in such a way that he has had to adopt the behaviour of the opposite gender to survive. He will give up the fight and begin to imitate the parent that was previously a rival and so affirm his identity.

However, parents who have unsatisfactory relationships may seek to encourage the child in his fantasies partly to bolster their own egos and partly to cause mischief between themselves and their partners. This situation may become very frightening for the child who fears that he may actually win. The reality of defeating a parent will make him feel guilty and unable to cope.

This situation may arise if, for example, a boy's father dies. If the boy had fantasied that he wished his father dead, the reality of the wish coming true is likely to make him very afraid of his powerfulness and very wary about expressing initiative in the future. His mother may compound the problem by saying 'Now you will have to be the man of the house' and may even take the boy to bed with her from apparently reasonable motives that they may comfort each other. This, however, may have the effect of making too close a bond between mother and son which will have strong sexual over-tones, particuarly if it occurs at this stage of genital awareness. The boy may find future relationships with other girls never quite as satisfying as this early sexual relationship with his mother and may well continue to live with his mother throughout his life. He will probably experience a great deal of trauma when she dies as he will not have allowed himself to become a separate person.

Sibling Rivalry

The birth of another child will have an effect on the existing children as it changes their position in the family, and therefore changes how members of the family relate to them. The greatest effect seems to be on the first-born at the birth of the second child, particularly if the first-born is passing through the genital stage (Lowe, 1972).

The conflicts and rivalries experienced in this period will be increased by the birth of the baby. The child may see the baby as brought in because he himself is causing so much trouble, or is not good enough. After all, if he were good enough his parents would not want another baby when they already have him. The birth may add to the sense of inadequacy that is very prevalent at this stage and the care and attention quite necessarily shown to the baby may cause the child to regress to an earlier stage in the hope of gaining the same attention for himself. It is quite usual for the child to become aggressive towards the baby. This may result in actual harm being done to the baby or, if the child feels too guilty to show how he feels, he may become over-loving and protective to the baby, in order to mask his true feelings.

Sexual Abuse

Sexual abuse of children at any age will have an effect on their developing sexuality, but may have the greatest effect if it occurs during the genital stage when the child is sensitive to its sexual feelings.

One form of sexual abuse often strongly denied by the child's parents is what could be called sexual overstimulation. This is when the parent of the opposite sex continues to touch the genitals of the child long after it is strictly necessary. The parent may call it 'Making sure that he is really clean' – but it will involve sexual handling over a long period of time. Tickling, which has sadistic as well as sexual overtones, may be common in a family and will produce the same effect, overstimulating the sexual feelings of the child. He is unable to discharge his feelings and may remain tense and irritable and be preoccupied with this sexual touching to the exclusion of other forms of activity.

A more severe form of sexual abuse is found in families with, as a rule, girls being more abused than boys (Renvoise, 1982). Father, brothers, grandfathers or uncles may be involved in the abuse. This sexual abuse may range from creeping into the child's bedroom to touch her genitals, to requiring the child to masturbate the abuser, to attempted rape. While this last incident is often thought of as the most shocking, if it is an isolated incident that is not blown up out of all proportion by the child's parents, it may cause less harm to the child's sexual development than continuing sexual incidents which lead to a conspiracy between the child and the abuser. The child's sexual feelings will be aroused; indeed she may have been the seducer. She is likely to feel flattered by the extra attention and older children may blackmail the abuser in order to gain extra favours. She may not want the sexual activity to stop.

However, guilt is experienced by the child and is compounded by the abuser who invariably warns the child to say nothing. An older child may be aware that if she reports the abuse, her father may go to prison. Renvoise (1982) suggests that in many cases the child's mother colludes in the sexual abuse. This may be because she was abused when a child and feels unable to stop history repeating itself or because she is glad that her husband's sexual attention is being diverted on to someone else. Indeed, she may deliberately leave the child and father in the house together. If the child does say anything to her then she is likely to dismiss the suggestion. Children in this situation, as they get older, appear to forgive their fathers, but not their mothers.

Sexual abuse may have two effects. If the abuse was not too frightening, then sexual feelings in later relationships may not be as arousing when compared with these earlier experiences. Or, if the degree of guilt is very great, it may lead to a suppression of all memory of the incident in order to suppress the anxiety of the sexual feelings. In later relationships, the arousal of sexual feelings will bring about an instant blocking of those feelings in order to protect the memory of the earlier incident. In dealing with sexual problems in adults, it may be necessary to help the patient to become aware of the sexual feelings of the earlier incidents.

An increasing problem area, with second marriages becoming common, is that of the stepfather, for whom the incest taboo does not exist. Another common area of abuse is by other adults when the child is away on holiday alone, or goes to stay with friends. This should be suspected in children who become disturbed or naughty on return from such visits. The child may be naughty because he is angry with his parents for allowing it to happen, or because he feels guilty for enjoying it and feels he should be punished.

Clues may be given at home or in school, such as drawing or writing stories. Teachers who are shocked by such ideas are not helping the child. An example is given by the NSPCC of a child of this age at school who drew a picture of a man with a very long erect penis with a dripping end – which she had labelled 'snot'. The headmistress sent for the child and threatened her with punishment if she ever drew such a disgusting thing again. But did the head-mistress really believe that the child could draw such a thing if she had not experienced it?

Pains in the lower abdomen in children often indicate general anxiety but may also indicate specific anxiety regarding sexual abuse.

7   7–12 YEARS

This stage involves a much longer time span than the previous three stages and broadly corresponds to primary schooling. Here the child's main focus and preoccupation is with his school life. In fact, school life often spills over into home life in the form of homework and school activities which are mirrored as play at home. He has moved from preoccupation with his family into the larger group of school and often into other group activities such as Brownies or Cubs, where again the emphasis is on training.

The sexuality of the genital stage becomes secondary to other interests and this stage is described by Freud as a period of latency. If the child has successfully negotiated the previous stage in which identification with the parent of the same sex has taken place and the Oedipal conflicts have been resolved, then the child will tend to play with other children of the same sex and will not need at this stage to test out his masculinity or femininity.

The child becomes enthusiastic to learn about the world and how it works and in doing so in school becomes involved in mastering social skills, conforming rather than asserting his independence. School, therefore, is a place for learning how to behave in society as well as for gaining knowledge. Other stages may be more relevant to developing the sexuality of the future adult, nevertheless, gaining knowledge and acquiring social skills will affect how that child will relate to others as an adult.

Knowledge

This is the age at which the child wants to learn about himself and anything else around him in his world. As he is not sexually and emotionally involved with the opposite sex, this is the time that sex education could be formally introduced at school, with emphasis on the facts about human growth and development, intercourse, reproduction and childbirth. Information could be given about the expected development of the child's body into that of an adolescent, information about periods, wet dreams and masturbation.

Children cover the same ground many times in the process of

47

learning, each time taking in that which is seen as relevant, building on previous information in order to reach a greater understanding of what is being studied. Information given now about sex could be built on the earlier information given when the child first looked at books with his mother. (See Chapter 9).

The other aspect of gaining knowledge is the development of the child's sense of achievement, of his worth in relation to other children. Great emphasis is placed on this in schools in the form of stars, grades and prizes. A child who becomes aware that he is not as clever as other children may develop into an adult who is lacking in self-esteem. This will affect how he relates to others. Even play at school may be structured in the same way with prowess in games being rewarded. Sometimes being good at games can make up for poor scholarship, but a child who is good at neither may feel very inferior.

Social skills

The acquisition of knowledge in school leads to a sense of achievement and usefulness, whereas the other aspect of school, that of working together in groups, develops a sense of belonging.

The child will have to learn to submerge his individuality and to conform to the needs of the group. There is usually a subtle shift from needing to observe the values of the parents to observing the values of peers at school. If there is a great difference and the child feels insecure, he may appear to be two people. An example of this is when the child speaks with one accent and behaves in one way at home and speaks with another accent and behaves differently at school. This may result in great conflict for the child, who may be reluctant to bring friends home or have his parents visit the school.

The ability to conform may be prevented by individual characteristics that make the child stand out from the rest. Difference in physical size is very important, although probably not as important as in the next stage, adolescence. Accent, parents' occupations, financial status reflected in the way the child dresses, colour, and even an unusual name can affect how well the child is accepted into the group.

Experience of relating to others at school will affect the ease with which an adult relates to others and so provides for himself opportunities for meeting a sexual partner.

8   12–19 YEARS

This span of years completes the child's transition from dependence to independence. Although the child is capable of a full physical sexual relationship during this time, by and large he is still economically dependent on his parents and so not a separate person. Consequently, this stage is considered under sexual and emotional development rather than in the section on adult sexuality.

Freud labelled this stage the genital period and the child is usually known as a teenager or adolescent. Adolescence is, however, a comparatively recent phenomena. In the past, the onset of physical maturity coincided with economic independence so that there was no conflict. In some cultures the separation from parents takes place with early marriage and this, therefore, provides for a legitimate satisfaction of the sex drive. Various initiation ceremonies mark the transition from childhood to adulthood so that the child is clear what role is expected at each stage. Even the change from short pants to long trousers in a boy or putting her hair up for a girl was recognised as a step across the threshold into adulthood. When marriage was not economically possible then strong religious views and chaperoning kept the sexual drive under control.

However, by the increase in the school leaving age and the onset of earlier sexual maturity (possibly because of better nutrition) a large gap has grown between the two, giving rise to a group of young people who have the potential for sexual activity without the corresponding economic independence. The decline in the influence of religion and the increasing influence of advertising and the media have contributed to the uncertainties of the adolescent who is urged to try everything in his search for identity. For most adolescents, this process is completed by the time they are about 19, yet for students in Higher Education, such as at University, this process may be delayed as striving for academic achievement takes priority. These young people may well go through the rebellion and striving for identity in their early twenties even though their bodies matured much earlier.

The changes that take place over this period may be described in terms of physical changes and a search for identity; of becoming a separate, sexual person.

Physical Change

This is a period of extensive physical change – both externally and internally in that physiological processes such as menstruation and the production of semen begin.

Growth

The maximum growth spurt for girls is at about 12 years and for boys at about 14 years. However, the rate of growth is quite uneven. Hands and feet become adult size before the body and arms and legs become longer, which leads to ungainly walking and a tendency to trip up and become clumsy. When this rapid change in size takes place, the previous perception of one's body is no longer true and uncertainty of movement will result.

Growth is stimulated by the growth hormone produced by the pituitary gland and regulated by somatostatin from the hypothalamus. The cortex of the adrenal gland produces androgens which also stimulate growth. Growth is complete when the epiphyseal plates in the long bones are finally calcified into bone. This is influenced by oestrogen in girls and testosterone in boys. It has been suggested that there is a link between tall, willowy girls and a late onset of menstruation, and it is also possible that boys who continue to grow well into their twenties have a lower than normal testosterone level.

There has also been concern lest giving the contraceptive pill, which contains oestrogen, to girls of 14 or 15 will close their epiphyseal plates prematurely and so restrict growth. However, no evidence of this has been found.

Puberty

This is the name given to the maturation of the reproductive system. This maturation usually occurs two years earlier in girls than boys, within a range of 9–16 years, with average age of menstruation being 12–13 years. It occurs in boys within a range of 10–18 years with the average age of first seminal emissions being 14–15 years (Tanner, 1971).

As with the growth hormone, the pituitary gland is the initiator, regulated by releasing factors from the hypothalmus. Follicle stimulating hormone and luteinizing hormone from the pituitary influences the ovaries in girls and the testes in boys – these are the target organs for these hormones.

In girls the ovaries are stimulated by the FSH and LH to produce ova and also to produce oestrogen, a hormone which causes secondary sex characteristics to develop. Often the first sign of the onset of puberty is the appearance of breast buds together with downing over the symphysis pubis and a rounding of the hips.

Subsequently, coarse, curly pubic hair forms on the mons in the shape of an inverted triangle, followed by the growth of axillary hair. The uterus enlarges and the endometrium develops under the influence of oestrogen and progesterone, also secreted by the ovary. The vagina, labia and clitoris develop. There is a white vaginal secretion occurring before the first menstruation. The first menstruation is called the menarche and it is common for the first menstrual cycles to be irregular before settling into an average 28–30 day cycle (Tanner, 1971). The first cycles are not indicative that conception can now occur, as ovulation may not have taken place, nor may the endometrium be able to support a pregnancy.

In boys, the testes are stimulated by the FSH and LH to produce sperm and also to produce testosterone, a hormone which influences the sperm production and is responsible for the development of the secondary sex characteristics. The penis becomes longer and with a greater circumference and there is an increase in size of the testes and scrotum, the skin of which becomes reddened and coarsened. As with girls, down may grow over the symphysis pubis.

Later, this hair will coarsen and become curly and change from an inverted triangle to extend up to the umbilicus. The axillary and facial hair develops next, but chest and other body hair may not develop until the age of twenty or over. As the prostate and seminal vesicles mature, emissions of semen begin, either induced by masturbation or occurring spontaneously during sleep – nocturnal emissions or wet dreams, which may be accompanied by vivid sexual dreams. However, the semen is infertile at this stage (Tanner, 1971). The penis, testes and scrotum continue to grow and the semen then contains live, mature sperm. The voice breaks as the larynx enlarges. The sweat glands are stimulated in both male and female, giving rise to body odours and skin problems such as acne.

Adapting to Change

The response to these changes in body image may be that of pleasure; that at last one is growing up. Some girls insist on their mothers buying a bra almost before they have anything to put in one and will wear, if allowed, shoes that are more suitable for the dance floor than for school.

Others may dread the onset of puberty; being ill-prepared and insecure, they may wish that they could maintain the status quo and not grow up. Parents' attitudes to growing up will influence this. A father who sees his daughter as 'daddy's girl' may well resent her emerging adult sexuality and fear competitors. The daughter who sees his displeasure, may indeed want to remain 'daddy's girl'. Anorexia nervosa in girls may be part of a complex reaction to not wanting to grow up (Crisp, 1980).

Menstruation being so much more dramatic than anything boys go through can either be seen as a blessing, as the gateway to womanhood, or, as it is often called, 'a curse'. The attitude of the girl's mother will influence how the girl sees it. If the girl has not been told anything, then to find herself apparently bleeding to death, can be a very frightening experience. To have thrust at her a packet of sanitary towels and be told this will happen once a month and that she might as well get used to it, is not very helpful. Mothers may go even further and give dire warnings about not getting pregnant and admonish 'Keep away from boys who will only take advantage of you'.

These sorts of experience will affect the emerging sexuality of the girl and how confident she feels in the acceptability of her body. A nice description of menstruation was given by a friend of mine to her five-year-son: 'The part of the body where the baby grows, makes food for the baby, hoping each month that it will have a baby to feed. When that does not happen, the food comes away so that new food can be made each month.' Her son will probably never remember being told that, but his attitude towards menstruation in girls will have been influenced by a mother who saw fit to explain natural bodily functions in a caring way.

Boys do not seem to attach the same importance to wet dreams or nocturnal emissions, although some of them say that it is embarrassing for them to wake up in a wet, sticky bed which may evoke memories of messing themselves as a child. Also they may worry that their mother might know. Wet dreams may evoke memories of punishment for masturbation and, if the boy is fearful of adulthood, then anything that demonstrates to him that he is on the brink of it will be unwelcome.

Those who do welcome the changes may be seen removing their emerging facial hair with a razor long before it is necessary, in an attempt to be seen as grown up. Boys seem to be far more preoccupied with the size of their penises than with other sexual aspects of their bodies and will compare size in the lavatories. Boys have to suffer the lack of control both of their voice, which in the breaking stage may be totally unpredictable, and the spontaneous erection of their penis. They may suffer agonies in the presence of a girl, fearing that she may have noticed it.

Adolescents become very self-conscious, imagining always that people are observing and judging every move. Their clumsiness may produce feelings of humiliation that they can behave in such a way. They become preoccupied with being the same as everyone else and dress according to their peer groups. The developmental changes are watched for in friends and compared with their own. Difference in size of anything, height, breasts, penis, will cause great concern. The boy who develops late seems to be most at risk from feeling different (Hamachek, 1973). As girls develop about two years earlier, he will be a loser in the competition for girlfriends and probably in sports competitions too and may suffer a permanent blow to his self-esteem as a result.

As well as the physical changes, the hormonal changes seem to influence the mood of the adolescent. The chemical balance of the body may be disturbed, producing, in some cases, transient almost psychotic changes. The adolescent may be subjected to severe swings of mood, from elation to despair, for no apparent reason, and his feelings may well be totally incomprehensible to himself as well as to his parents.

The Search for Identity

It would hardly be surprising if the adolescent had an identity crisis based on his changing shape and physiology alone, but as well as coming to terms with these changes, and the implications of the changes, he must complete his education, get a job, move out of his home and find a sexual partner, all over a span of a few years. However, the most pressing question for him to answer is, 'Who and what am I?'

In an attempt to answer this question the adolescent identifies with older members of the same sex, maybe a teacher or youth leader, and may try to be like them. However, eventually the adolescent becomes dissatisfied with his model and may discard it, keeping only those bits of the adult's personality which seem to fit. Other people will then be chosen and the process repeated.

Pop stars or film stars are frequently chosen for models, both for the individual adolescent and for his peer group as a whole. It may be part of the group pressure to conform to liking one particular pop star or group. If the adolescent has difficulty in choosing people with whom to interact and on whom to model his behaviour, then he may live in a fantasy world. This is much less helpful to him in his search for identity. Real models demonstrate all too readily that they are not perfect and not exactly like the adolescent, whereas a fantasy model can be made into whatever the adolescent wishes.

The adolescent may choose different ways to behave (perhaps using as models people he knows) and in those roles interact with others to test out 'Is this me?' Parents who observe this rapid shift in personality may become very confused and concerned at this choice of apparently unsuitable lifestyles and friends. The reassurance that parents need at this stage is that nothing is fixed yet in the adolescent and, if left alone, most of the strange behaviour will go away.

The adolescent seems to see everything in black and white, as right or wrong; he tends to become idealistic, angry at the compromises of life, moralistic, and may become attached to 'lost causes', identifying with someone else that they admire who is involved in the movement.

In this search for identity, the outward sign to the parents may be that of rebellion. However, this may be the visible part of his drive to separate. At the end of his search for identity, having discarded the models that do not fit, the emerging adult may resemble his parents in some ways and yet not in others. Some adolescents whose parents are very strict and who will not tolerate any rebellion, may end up frightened to separate and with little identity of their own. These people may have to go through the adolescent period much later in life.

The opposite of this is the adolescent who is fearful of the smothering of his parents and who has to fight very hard to be a separate individual. He may consciously adopt a lifestyle the complete opposite of his parents'. Similarly, children of very trendy parents may have to become very conforming and straight-laced in order to rebel. Parents who do not provide any boundaries for their children may find that they have delinquent adolescents who have to produce increasingly rebellious behaviour in order to find the boundaries they need to react against. Adolescents who find the whole thing far too difficult may opt out by taking drugs, alcohol or sniffing glue.

If an adolescent suffers a long-term illness or permanent disability at the time of his life when he is searching for an identity and learning to make relationships with the opposite sex, this can be a serious setback to his development.

Nurses caring for such patients should realise the need these adolescents have for support and the stresses they may face in modifying their expectations for the future – perhaps drastically. The patients may fear that they will never be acceptable and that they will miss the opportunities for the trial and error in relationships that is generally accepted in adolescence. They may arrive home from hospital to find that they have lost their friends and have few social skills with which to make new relationships.

In order to help to keep the patient in the mainstream of life, nurses need to be prepared to give support and encouragement to these adolescents to dress up and use make-up (if appropriate) and to maintain their interaction with other young people.

The Search for a Sexual Life

There has been a general trend both in Britain and America for adolescents to have sexual intercourse at an early age (Tom McGlew, Department of Social Science, Edinburgh University, and Chilman, 1978), and it is estimated that one in five adolescent girls become pregnant in the first month of sex. The average age of childbearing has fallen, nevertheless, fewer adolescents are marrying as a result of the pregnancy. What is happening is that the illegitimacy rate is rising (80 per cent of all conceptions under 20 years in England and Wales are outside marriage) and also the abortion rate is rising (one-third of teenage pregnancies end in abortion), although it is still less than in other countries. The girls who do marry when pregnant, seem to be working-class girls (88 per cent of births that are conceived before marriage are to working-class girls). Chilman (1979) found that in America a substantially greater proportion of blacks had illegitimate births and were less likely to have an abortion.

The search for a sexual relationship tends to follow a pattern. In the early teens, 'crushes' on older people of the same sex are common. There are also close, sometimes physical relationships involving holding hands or walking arm in arm with friends of the same sex of about the same age. This physical contact between girls is not often commented on as it is fairly acceptable as part of women's caring role for them to touch. However, boys who show the same outward physical demonstration of caring to each other are often seen as deviant.

The middle teens is a period of experimentation with many different partners of the opposite sex, not always fully sexual. At first boys and girls may go around together in groups, but gradually couples break away on their own. This is when the double standard of sexual permissiveness arises. Boys are allowed, even encouraged, to have sexual partners before marriage, but girls are supposed to be virgins on marriage. This double standard does still exist, but modified so that virginity on marriage is now seen by most as unrealistic. However, this conflict affects how boys and girls see their early relationships. Boys are encouraged by their peers to 'collect scalps' of girls with whom they have had intercourse, whereas peer groups of girls may not see this as an acceptable practice for girls. Girls who advertise the fact that they are indulging in sex at this stage – aged 14–15 – will still tend to be seen as 'tarts' or 'sluts' by their contemporaries. This conflict of girls having to be 'good' and boys experienced, is usually solved by boys using the willing 'tarts' to gain experience or boasting of their sexual adventures even if they have not managed to acquire the experience.

In later teens, more settled relationships are established with the opposite sex and these will often include sexual intercourse.

The adolescent's search for sexual identity may be very threatening to the parent's sexual life. When an emerging nubile woman, without wrinkles, grey hair and bags under her eyes, suddenly appears in their household, the mother may feel the threat of competition again for the father and in a form far more likely to succeed than in the Oedipal stage. If the mother is still very attractive herself, she may enter into competition with her daughter for the daughter's boyfriends. The adolescent in either case may thus have difficulty in coming to terms with her sexuality. The position of boys in relation to their father may well mirror this – with father in competition, showing off to his son's girlfriends.

The sexual functioning of the parents may be affected if they worry about the adolescents hearing them making love. This may lead to impotence in the man or a loss of sexual response in a woman. Unresolved conflicts of the parents may force them to react over-harshly to the sexuality of their children.

Contraception

Unfortunately, knowing the facts about conception and contraception does not seem to influence the use of contraception when experimenting with sex.

A survey in Britain (Tom McGlew, unpublished) into the use of contraception at the first sexual experience of 16–19 year-olds showed that 37 per cent used the sheath, 10 per cent used withdrawal, 8 per cent were on the pill and 47 per cent used nothing. I suspect that a survey of sexual experience under this age would show an even lower use of contraception. In America Zelnik and Kantner (1977) surveyed women between the ages of 15 and 19 and found that 25 per cent of women had never used contraception. Experience in family planning clinics shows that the vast majority of adolescents requesting contraception are already having intercourse, many of them previously unprotected. However, Brook Advisory Clinics in Scotland found that approximately one-third of the requests for the pill occur before intercourse has taken place (Health Bulletin, May 1982). This may be because Brook clinics were specifically set up to meet the needs for contraception of adolescents and those under 25 years of age.

There may be several difficulties in accepting the use of contraception. In order for girls to take the pill, it requires a conscious decision that they wish to have sex and needs a visit to the doctor. It may also involve waiting until the pill is effective. This premeditation in the confused moral world of the girl, may be seen as showing that she is ready to have sex and is, therefore, 'easy'. If the girl has not accepted her sexuality, she will not see intercourse as acceptable unless it is not premeditated or she gets 'carried away'. She will also have difficulty in accepting that it will happen again and so make no future preparation. At this stage she is not prepared to take responsibility for her sexual feelings and prefers a seduction, for it to be out of her control.

A boy who carries sheaths or rubbers in his pocket, apart from to show to other boys at school as evidence of his sexual exploits, will be seen by girls as only wanting them for sex. The boy may hope that the girl is on the pill, so that he does not have to worry, but if he finds that she is on the pill he may think that she is 'anybody's'.

With this difficulty in accepting girls' sexuality by both boys and girls, it is hardly surprising that contraception is not used.

A further difficulty is that the legal age for sex with a girl is 16 years. Consequently, it is difficult for girls under that age to ask for contraception. It is only exceptionally mature girls who will pluck up courage to do so and experience in clinics has shown that even if on their first visit they are not prepared for their parents to be informed, by the time they return for their three month check many have at least told their mothers. It would be interesting to speculate on how much the Law's forbidding under-age intercourse actually affects the rate of intercourse under 16 years. I wonder whether those who would deny contraceptive services and advice to the under 16s really understand the problems of adolescent sexuality.

The failure of adolescent girls to use contraception can be explained in some cases by an unconscious wish to have a baby. If a girl has had an unsatifactory childhood, has achieved little at school, then one way for her to be noticed is to become pregnant (Specht and Craig, 1982). Feeling unloved herself, she thinks that a baby will give her the love she needs, little realising that a baby also needs frequent feeding and changing, and often cries. Girls seem to be unable to see beyond having this baby to the difficulties that lie ahead.

The development of the individual from conception to young adulthood has now been covered, albeit by dividing the years into ages and stages. It should be stressed, however, that these divisions are somewhat arbitrary; they are merely a way of considering the factors influencing development in a systematic way, each at the time at which it seems to be most relevant.

The question of sex education as a positive way of influencing the development of the individual will be discussed in the next chapter, which to some extent recapitulates what has gone before in this part of the book.

9   SEX EDUCATION

Although most people seem to agree that there should be sex education, there is a continuing debate about what it should consist of and by whom it should be carried out. Does it consist of showing children what the body looks like and telling them how it works? Should it include how to have intercourse and should the subject be dealt with in the wider context of relationships, feelings, responsibilities and moral issues?

Sometimes what is little more than a lesson in biology is called sex education, but my favourite definition of sex education comes from James Hemmings (1971):

> We start with the egocentric, mother-dependent infant. We seek to end with a confident, passionate, sensitive, tender, considerate, socially responsible adult. Whatever helps growth so that the one is gradually transformed into the other, may be properly regarded as sex education.

There is no such thing as no sex education. The child who says 'I did not receive any sex education from my parents' is, in fact, saying that he received a negative input about sex. The fact that parents never say anything about sex is in itself sex education – the message being, 'We do not talk about things like that.'

In my view, sex education should be positive, started by the parents when the child is old enough to look at picture books and to ask simple questions about his body and continued throughout his social life by both parents *and* teachers.

Several books are available and suitable for the 3–5 year-old pre-school child. The books contain pictures and simple words about mummy and daddy, with full frontal nude colour pictures of parents lying together and deciding that they want a baby, pictures of the baby growing in the womb and, in some, pictures of the birth. Children are usually fascinated at this age by these stories and want to hear them again and again.

The advantage for parents who are worried about how they will approach sex education for their children, is that introduced at this age and in this way, they do not have to worry in the future about the best time to talk about the facts of life. The child will grow up knowing that it is acceptable to talk about bodies and the scene will be set for the child to ask more complicated questions when they occur to him. However, a child's questions should be answered in a simple way, giving no more information than is asked for. The child who asks 'Why does daddy have a beard?' may be only comparing him with the man next door rather than asking for a lecture on the secondary sex characteristics. Sex education in the early years should be treated as the beginning of a learning spiral, with information being given, digested, consolidated by other questions and experience – all leading to a gradually increased understanding.

Primary Education

When the child is in primary school, one of the many projects that the child could undertake would be to follow a willing mum-to-be through her pregnancy. Children are interested in weighing and measuring and charting at this stage. The baby as it grows could be brought into school to have its development charted as well. This would link with television programmes such as 'Merry-go-round' about conception, birth and development. However, to be effective it must be recognised that the teachers need to feel comfortable with their own sexuality so that they can answer without embarrassment questions that will arise after these programmes. Parents too, need to be involved and should be given the opportunity of seeing the films before the children are shown them.

Teachers may worry that in a class of mixed ability, some children will be ready for information whilst others are not. However, it is generally believed that a child will pick up what he is ready for and reject the rest. Girls and boys should be taught together if possible rather than being segregated – otherwise it will emphasise the fact that this is special.

I believe that the pre-puberty schoolchild should be in possession of the facts of life – menstruation, wet dreams, growth of hair, change of voice and body shape – so that these can be anticipated as a milestone on the way to growing up. I would prefer to see this information being given in the final year of primary school, whilst the child is in a safe, known atmosphere. It is important to give the information before the occurrence of the hormonal changes which bring on not only the physical changes but also the emotional changes. Once this happens the child's response to information becomes subjective rather than objective.

Secondary Education

It is necessary for secondary school teachers to check what information has been given previously and, perhaps more important, to check what has been received – some children may not have 'heard' previous information.

Ths adolescent has several needs relating to sex education: the need for information about contraception, venereal disease and other health-related subjects; the acceptance of his sexuality; the opportunity to discuss with his peers his attitudes to sex, his relationship with parents, teachers and friends of both sexes. A school has an important function in providing a framework within which adolescents may test out their perception of what is right for them.

Generally speaking and unfortunately, the students in any one school do not always have equal opportunities for sex education. Middle and lower achievers may have room made in their timetable for formal sex education. This may be partly to pass the time and partly because these students often demonstrate their emerging sexuality more overtly. Indeed, the staff may fear that they will have a pregnancy on their hands if they do not do something about it. On the other hand, academic students rarely have room in their timetables for anything other than academic subjects and, unless one of the subjects happens to be biology, they will miss out on the basic facts of life as well as on the peer group discussions.

Nurses may become involved with sex education of schoolchildren when the teacher, who may feel inadequate in handling the subject, requests help from the school nurse, health visitor or family planning nurse. Teachers are very sensitive to parents' pressures on them if they become too daring about sex education and they may, therefore, feel that a health visitor who talks about contraception along with other health matters, will cause less trouble than asking a family planning nurse into the school to talk about contraception.

These requests raise the issue of who is better qualified to give the talks – the experts who have the most up-to-date information or those who are expert at teaching and developing discussion. One point put forward in favour of outsiders leading discussion groups is that students might be more likely to speak freely with someone from outside the school whom they will not have to face the next day. The argument for the subject being handled by teachers is that the teachers can build a relationship with the students that will continue, as questions about sex will not just stop when the outsider finishes her talk. Perhaps a compromise would be the school nurse who has already made relationships with the teachers and students.

Certainly outsiders coming into school emphasises that sex is different and, perhaps, a more constructive role for the experts is in training teachers and parents who are going to give the sex education. Just as the parents' attitudes to their own sexuality affects the way they give sex education to their children, the attitude of teachers will affect how well they handle the subject in school. Indeed, how they relate to the different sexes in an ordinary class in sex education.

Although there has been an increasing awareness of the need for sex education both by parents and by schools, the present situation is far from satisfactory. Research by Yvonne Bostock and Douglas Leather (1982) into the attitude to sexual behaviour and contraception of young people between the ages of 16 and 20 and to get their views on the value of mass media on these subjects' showed that:

> The results indicated that communication is poor between schools and young people and between parents and children; that practical information is lacking; and that society subjects young people to a multitude of conflicting pressures and expectations.
>
> They also indicated that mass media campaigns have only a limited role to play, as the subject is complex and concerns the individual coming to terms with the moral, religious and social implications of being a sexually mature person. Any real change in attitude can only be achieved by a broader approach involving schools, parents and the whole of society.

Sex Education in Hospitals or Institutions

Apart from assisting with sex education in schools, nurses should be aware that children in long-term hospital or institutional care will have a need for sex education. These children will miss the opportunities for informal sex education which occur during day-to-day living at home. These include seeing male and female naked bodies, learning about male and female roles, being told by their parents about growing up and sexual development, and learning to make relationships.

Thus the nurse, as part of her responsibility for total patient care, may need to plan a more formal approach to sex education – even if she is not the person who will carry this out. It may be something which is undertaken by a playleader, nursery nurse, teacher, or by health educators from the Health Education Department. Regardless of who undertakes the sex education, provision needs to be made for books to be available, perhaps films to be shown and discussion to be held – in a similar way to the approach to the subject in many schools.

It is difficult enough for any child to forge a sexual identity, but a child who is forced to be continually dependent because of illness, whose emerging sexuality may be seen as a threat to both his parents and to his nurses, has a much more difficult task in making relationships on equal terms. He needs practical, positive help from his carers.

Suggested Further Rading for Part II

Dallas, Dorothy M, *Sex Education in School and Society* (National Foundation for Educational Research England and Wales, 1972).

English, O.S. and Pearson, G.H.J., *Emotional Problems of Living,* 3rd edition (Allen and Unwin, 1965).

Lowe, Gordon, R., *The Growth of Personality _ from Infancy to Old Age* (Pelican, 1972)

Specht, Riva and Craig, Grace J., *Human Development _ A Social Work Perspective* (Prentice Hall, 1982).

PART III

ADULT SEXUALITY

The previous section dealt with the factors influencing the sexual and emotional development of the child as he progresses towards adulthood. However, it would be wrong to suggest that at about the age of 19 years, maturation is complete and that no further development takes place. As far as physical development is concerned, the body continues to change, and although brain development is completed, the association areas of the brain are capable of continuing to make connecting links between new and old material, thus enabling learning to take place.

Emotional growth continues with each individual developing at his own rate. This is governed partly by that individual's preparedness to allow new experiences to influence him and partly by the availability of new experiences.

This part of the book is concerned with the broad stages of adult development until old age, and with the normal facets of life which may influence adult sexuality.

However, before looking at factors which may influence adult sexuality, it is useful to consider how the sexual organs are structured, and how this relates to the way that they function. Each person is constrained by the way that his body works, and a greater understanding of this will help both the nurse and the patient to realise what is possible, and what is unrealistic.

In this account, emphasis will be placed on the particular aspects of
the sexual organs which are related to sexual functioning. This
account should not therefore be taken as a full description of the
male and female sexual and reproductive system.

Female

The Vulva

This is the external part of a woman's sexual organs. It consists of
two thick outer lips covered with hair, called the labia majora.
These lips are joined to the pad of fat over the symphysis pubis,
which is also covered with hair, and called the mons veneris.

Figure 10.1: External Appearance of the Female

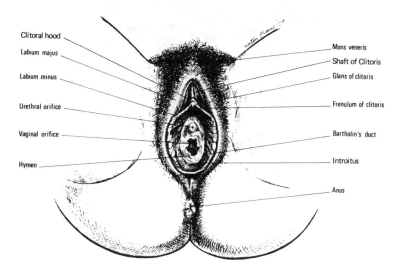

Inside the outer lips are the inner lips or labia minora. These are
hairless and join together over the clitoris to form the clitoral hood.

Towards the anus they join to form the fourchette, which is part of the perineum – a muscular body between the vagina and rectum (Figure 10.2).

Figure 10.2: Sagittal Section of the Female Pelvis

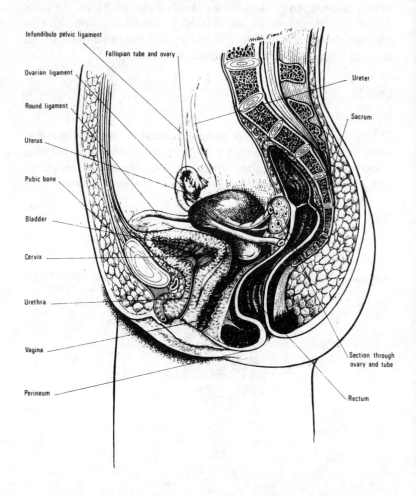

On parting the labia minora, the clitoris is seen within the fold of the hood. The clitoris consists of a glans – a tiny pea-like structure; and a shaft – which cannot be seen, only felt, running towards the mons, and feeling like a pencil lead (or with a stretch of the imagination, a tiny subcutaneous penis). These clitoral structures, as with most of the sexual organs, vary in size from person to person. They are extremely sensitive, particularly if touched directly without the area being lubricated. Below the clitoris, if lying on one's back, is the urethral opening, and below that, the opening to the vagina – the introitus.

Many women have never examined themselves in a mirror to see how they are made, and often have only a vague idea of where their clitoris is and are even less aware that they have a clitoral shaft, which is one of the important areas for sexual stimulation in the woman.

The Vagina

This consists of a tube, whose walls are in folds, allowing for distension, and which are approximately 8 cm long. From the outside, the vagina extends inwards towards the 'nob' of the cervix of the uterus, and the posterior fornix – the 'back pocket' of the vagina. The angle of the vagina frequently causes confusion for the insertion of tampons, the diaphragm and sometimes the penis, as both men and women expect that the vagina follows the general line of the body. This confusion may cause difficulties in intercourse if neither partner is quite sure about what angle the penis should be approaching at in order to penetrate. Diagrams such as in Figure 10.2 or a pelvic model are useful to demonstrate the angle of the vagina in relation to the body.

At the outer entrance to the vagina are two Bartholin's glands, with ducts leading into the vagina. Bancroft (1983) suggests that they contribute to vaginal lubrication after arousal has taken place.

Almost immediately inside the opening of the vagina is the hymen, which is a thin ring of tissue, perforated in the middle to allow the passage of blood during menstruation. Many people believe that the hymen remains intact throughout virginity and thus that absence of or damage to the hymen, indicates that intercourse has taken place. However, the hymen may be stretched or destroyed by the use of tampons or self exploration, and its presence or otherwise is no indicator of virginity or sexual experience.

Some people also believe that in her first intercourse a woman's hymen will rupture, causing pain and bleeding. Even is she has an intact hymen, this is not necessarily so – thus the idea of blood on the sheets on honeymoon being a sign of virginity is a myth. However, in some cultures the concept of virginity is very important, and, unless there is a strong medical reason, I do not believe that women should be examined vaginally if they have not had intercourse, unless they request it for reassurance that they are normal.

Continuing inside the vagina, after about 2 cm it passes through the levator ani muscles of the pelvic floor. A woman who is very anxious about a vaginal examination, or about intercourse, may tense these muscles involuntarily, making it impossible to examine her, or for her partner to penetrate. This condition is called 'vaginismus'.

The outer third of the vagina is well supplied with nerves; the inner two-thirds of the vagina is virtually non-sensitive and is much more elastic.

The vagina is lined with squamous epithelium and is surrounded by vascular spongy tissue, which is capable of being engorged with blood on sexual stimulation, in a similar way that the penis becomes erect by blood flowing into it. These tissues play an important part in the lubrication of the vagina which occurs as part of sexual arousal. Tissue fluid from the engorged tissues passes into the vagina in what Masters and Johnson (1966) describe as a sweating effect – drops of moisture appear all over the walls of the vagina. It was previously thought that the cervix contributed to the lubrication, but lubrication is unimpaired in women who have had a total hysterectomy (Bancroft, 1983).

The Uterus, Fallopian Tubes and Ovaries

The uterus consists of a body and a cervix or neck. The main concern regarding sexual functions is the position in which it lies. Normally it is anteverted as in Figure 10.2. Lying in this position it is quite clear of the posterior fornix, or 'back pocket' of the vagina into which the penis enters on intercourse. However, if the uterus is retroverted, and particularly if it is fixed in that position, it could be hit during intercourse, causing pain on deep penetration.

Attached to the uterus are the fallopian tubes, and lying in the broad ligament, near to the fimbriated ends of the tubes, are the ovaries. As far as sexual functioning is concerned, their importance is in the fact that they produce oestrogen, which is responsible for the development and maintenance of the secondary sexual characteristics, as well as the health of the lining of the vagina.

Male

The external genitalia of the male are more easily visible than in the female, and therefore seem to give rise to less fantasy, mystery and misunderstanding, apart from the aspect of size.

The Penis

The size of the unstimulated penis varies considerably from person to person, and bears little relationship to its size when erect. A man with a penis which is small when flaccid, will notice a proportionally greater lengthening than will a man with a penis which is large when flaccid (Masters and Johnson, 1966).

Concern about the size of the penis seems to be related to the presence of other sexual problems. Observations at school during puberty may be responsible for deep-seated fears of inequality, lack of self-esteem, and lack of confidence in the ability to perform and to be accepted sexually by a woman. Apart from the effect these concerns have on performance, the size of the penis bears little relationship to a man's ability to satisfy a woman sexually.

The penis consists of a shaft, arising from the base of the abdomen, and a head or glans. The abdomen at this point is covered with hair – which rises to a point at the level of the umbilicus – unlike in a woman, where the hair level is flat above the pubis. The penis itself is hairless, and the glans is covered, in an uncircumcised male, by a foreskin or prepuce. This foreskin may become retracted on erection, but certainly on intercourse (Figure 10.3).

Circumcision is the removal of the foreskin, either shortly after birth for religious reasons or because it is imperforated or later in life due to inflamation or stricture (phimosis). Circumcision is an essential feature of Judaism and is common practice in the United States of America, whereas it is not now common in Britain. This difference sometimes leads to partners in cross-cultural relationships having different expectations of what is the 'norm'. For example, an American woman may blame the failure of her British partner to have or maintain an erection on the fact that he has not been circumcised, as her previous experience of American men was probably that they had been circumcised, and she had never before experienced such a failure.

On the underside of the penis when hanging down, the foreskin is joined to the glans at the frenum. This area is the most sensitive part of the glans.

Figure 10.3: External Appearance of the Male

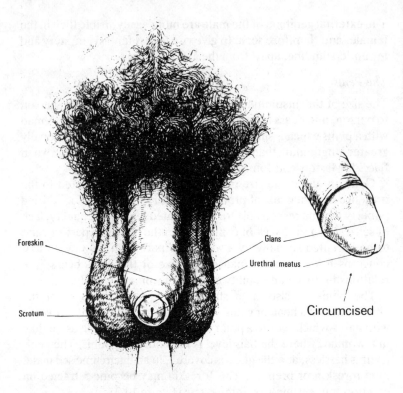

Foreskin

Scrotum

Glans

Urethral meatus

Circumcised

The shaft of the penis consists of two spongy structures called the corpora cavernosa on the upper surface and another spongy structure through which the urethra passes, on the lower surface of the penis. These structures run the length of the penis and become filled with blood (from the internal pudental artery, a branch of the internal iliac artery) when sexual arousal occurs – thus causing the erection of the penis. Constriction of this artery by atheroma or arteriosclerosis may affect the blood supply to the penis, and thus lead to erectile problems.

Muscles near the base of the penis are responsible for causing the ejaculation of seminal fluid.

The Scrotum and Testes

Hanging down below and behind the penis is the scrotum which contains the testes. These are external to the body, and are normally at a lower temperature, facilitating the production of sperm. One testicle usually hangs lower than the other. The skin of the scrotum is reddened and hairy and the testicles are painful if knocked.

Sperm, which are produced in the sertoli cells of the testes, are carried in the vas deferens to the urethra at the base of the bladder (Figure 10.4). Here they are joined by secretions from the seminal vesicles and prostate gland. Secretions from Cowper's gland during sexual arousal may cause fluid to be discharged from the penis before ejaculation; this amount may vary considerably and may contain sperm (Bancroft, 1983).

Figure 10.4: Sagittel Section of the Male Pelvis

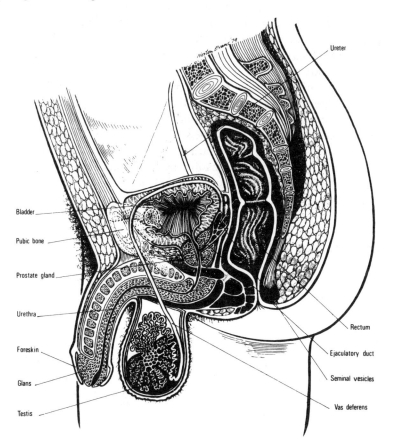

The other function of the testes is to produce testosterone from the intestitial cells. Although testosterone is involved in the production of sperm, it is not dependent on the production of sperm, thus a man with azospermia may have normal testosterone levels and normal sexual fuctioning.

The scrotum contains muscles which lift the testes in the scrotum during sexual arousal, and when the scrotum is exposed to unaccustomed cold.

Nerve Supply Involved in Sexual Response

The sensory fibres supplying male and female genitalia, lead to the 2nd and 3rd sacral roots of the spinal cord, in the pudendal nerve. Motor nerves from S4 supply muscles in the pelvis, perineum and penis. Sympathetic nerves from the thoracic and lumbar region, and parasympathetic nerves from S2, 3 and 4 supply the sexual organs (Bancroft, 1983). Their function will be considered when looking at sexual response.

In addition to the local nerve supply, which acts in a reflex arc through the spinal cord, centres in the brain, probably in the limbic system, are linked with sexual functioning. This area is mainly concerned with stimulation of the sexual response by the emotions, fantasy, the senses of smell, hearing, sight, and touch of other parts of the body; or with depression by fear, anxiety or distaste. Hormones and other chemicals, such as drugs, may influence the sex centres by stimulating or depressing sexual desire.

Other Areas of the Body

There are other parts of the body, in addition to the genitalia, that may be involved in sexual response. These areas may vary from person to person.

Breasts

In many people this is a sexually responsive area. The nipples become erect on sexual arousal in both men and women, and stimulation of the breasts alone may be sufficient, for some women, to produce an orgasm.

Anus

This may be stimulated by touching the outside, by penetration on anal intercourse, or by friction on the colon or penetration of the vagina.

Other areas of the body are highly specific to some people, and may be as important to them as part of their sexual arousal as are the genitalia to other people.

Kaplan (1979) divides sexual response into three phases, desire, excitement and orgasm.

Desire

Apart from suggesting that the desire phase of sexual response is controlled by the sex centres in the brain as described, little is known about the actual mechanism. Nevertheless, it is seen as a separate phase as patients may complain of failure of desire, even if their ability to be aroused and to have an orgasm is unimpaired. Similarly, a person may feel a strong desire for sex and yet have failure of arousal and orgasm.

Hormones which affect sexual desire are T_3 and T_4, FSH, LH, testosterone and prolactin. This latter hormone inhibits sexual desire quite markedly. Drugs such as Beta blockers, tranquillisers and antidepressants will also inhibit sexual desire. Alcohol, in small amounts, may increase desire, by lowering inhibitions of fear or guilt, however, since alcohol is basically a depressant, in larger amounts it may inhibit desire, or erectile function.

Excitement

The genital organs respond to stimuli from two sources – from the brain and from direct touch, through a spinal reflex. Either of these two types of stimulus may act on the genitals on its own, mainly through the parasympathetic nerve supply. However, they may be complementary, thus increasing the excitement, or antagonistic, with the central inhibition overriding local touch stimuli and leading to sexual failure (Figure 11.1).

It is important to note that sexual excitement does not rise at a steady rate, but rises in steps (Figure 11.2). This should be explained to patients experiencing difficulty in maintaining erection, as, if they sense a lessening in their erection, however temporarily, they may become anxious, thus activating the sympathetic nervous system which will then override their parasympathetic arousal

Figure 11.1: Interdependance of Stimuli to the Brain and the Genital Reflex

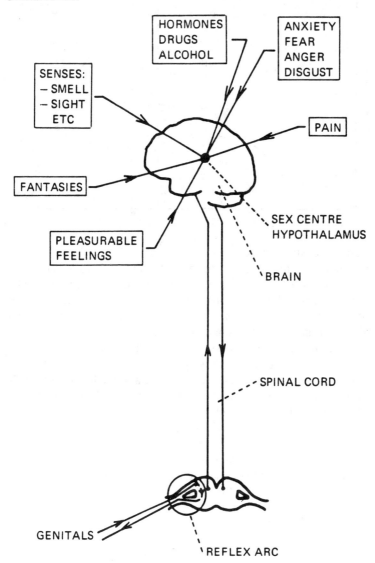

Figure 11.2: Pattern of Sexual Response

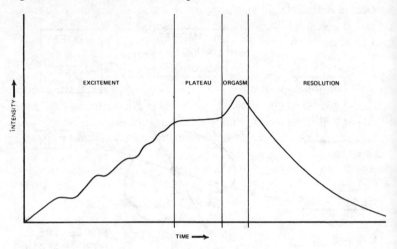

system, causing failure.

Once excitement begins, the main feature of this phase if that of vasocongestion, both of the genitals and of the body generally. Masters and Johnson (1966) describe this as a 'sex flush'. Other general effects in both sexes are increase in pulse, respiration and blood pressure and a tensing of muscles.

In women the vasocongestion leads to the labia minora becoming swollen and moist, so that they open slightly to reveal the introitus. The clitoris becomes enlarged and erect, and the lubrication of the vagina occurs. This is thought to be a transudate through the vagina walls due to the increased blood supply to the tissues surrounding the vagina. This lubrication is an early sign of arousal and the rate of lubrication or 'wetness' is greatest at the beginning of sexual response, reducing as sexual activity is prolonged.

Other features of arousal in women are erection of nipples, ballooning of the inner third of the vagina and lifting of the uterus from its normal position in the pelvis. This latter feature is impor- tant to women with a retroverted uterus. If intercourse takes place when the woman is sexually unstimulated, particularly if she is lying on her back, the thrusting of the penis may hit the uterus, causing pulling of the broad ligament in which the ovaries are situated, and causing pain. A suggestion to change the position of intercourse, or to make sure that the woman is sexually aroused before entry, may be sufficient to relieve this problem.

Vasocongestion in men leads to the penis becoming longer, thicker and erect. In addition, the scrotum lifts and becomes tense and the nipples become erect in 60 per cent of men (Masters and Johnson, 1966).

Plateau

This is the final part of the excitement stage. Pulse, respiration and blood pressure rise further, and vasocongestion is at its peak, causing in the woman what Masters and Johnson call an orgasmic platform – which is the swelling of the tissues surrounding the outer third of the vagina, which, in turn, gives extra stimulation to the penis. The penis secretes a few drops of fluid, probably from Cowper's gland, and the coronal ridge becomes fully distended and the testes become fully elevated.

Orgasm

Provided that the degree of stimulation of the clitoris or penis is sufficient, or an adequate amount of stimulation via the brain occurs, then the orgasmic reflex takes place, governed by the sympathetic nerve supply. There is often some degree of loss of consciousness and severe muscle spasm such as arching of the back, at the time of orgasm. As with the other stages, the sex centre in the brain may act against the genital stimulation, preventing the reflex from occurring.

In men, the orgasm takes place in two stages. The first stage is one of emission, when the semen collects in the urethra. Men may be able to recognise this stage as the point when they know that one or two further thrusts will lead to ejaculation and is often called the point of inevitability. The second stage is that of ejaculation, when the semen is expelled down the urethra, and out of the penis in spurts of approximately 0.8 second intervals initially (Masters and Johnson, 1966) caused by contraction of the penile muscles. During ejaculation the bladder is closed off from the urethra, at the inner sphincter, thus preventing the semen being forced into the bladder and preventing urination. However, sometimes following prostatectomy and in other diseases such as diabetes, this sphincter is damaged, causing retrograde ejaculation – when the semen is ejaculated into the bladder, giving a dry orgasm.

In women, because there is no semen to collect, it is generally accepted that orgasm is a one-stage operation; nevertheless, some women have reported to me that they can identify a stage of inevitability, where the sensations definitely change prior to orgasm. At orgasm, similar contractions of 0.8 second intervals occur in the outer third of the vagina. This may force out lubrication fluid, or previously deposited semen, giving rise to the suggestion that women have an ejaculation in the same way as men. The uterus also contracts, which can cause lower abdominal pain at the time of orgasm.

Resolution

After orgasm, the pulse, respiration and blood pressure quickly return to normal, and there is a general feeling of well being and relaxation. Men have what is called a refractory period during which they are unable to be restimulated. This may vary from a few seconds in a young man, to 24 hours in a man aged over 40 years; however, as with most things, this will vary from person to person. Older men, who may feel that there is something wrong with them and who may present with what they see as impotence, may be helped by explaining what is 'normal'.

Women generally do not have this refractory period and may be restimulated after orgasm, and go on to have further orgasms.

In this description of desire, excitement and orgasm, it is important to note that sexual response has a considerable subjective element that is impossible to quantify or describe. How people interpret the physiological process of arousal and orgasm will depend on what it means to them in emotional terms and will be influenced by their past experiences. In addition, the degree of arousal and the time taken to reach orgasm may vary considerably from person to person, and may also vary in the same person at different times.

Both men and women can experience sexual desire and excitement, and yet still experience pleasure, with a feeling of well being and relaxation afterwards, without having an orgasm. Many women, in particular, may experience a very enjoyable sexual relationship without ever having an orgasm, and this therefore should not be seen as a problem if the woman is happy and satisfied.

However, once the plateau stage has been reached, if orgasm does not occur, then both man and woman will feel very uncomfortable, tense and irritable, and this feeling will often take several hours to dissipate. Repeated frustration of this kind can become a problem.

ADULTHOOD

In the next three chapters adulthood has been divided into three periods: 20–40 years – young adulthood; 40–60 years – middle life; and 60 years onwards – old age. Although the life events described here occur to different people at different ages, and thus it is difficult to generalise, nevertheless I have attempted to discuss those events which affect sexual relationships, in the age group for which they seem to be the most appropriate.

Growth in the long bones may continue until around 25 years of age and body hair continues to develop in men. People of this age are generally at their peak of health. These years are concerned with finding a job, seeking a permanent sexual partner, getting married and having and raising children.

Work

Finding a job or pursuing a career may be more important to men than women, both from the point of view of finance and career development. Women, however, particularly if they have their children in their early twenties, will tend to be less concerned with a job than with raising a family unless there are strong financial or other reasons for not doing so.

Work seems to play an important part in a man's self-esteem. The traditional idea of the man as the breadwinner is very embedded in the stereotype of the masculine role, and anything such as un-employment, redundancy or job insecurity which threatens his role may well have an effect on how he sees himself as a man. If he becomes unsure of himself in the area of his work then this often affects his sexual functioning.

An ambitious man, provided that he can get a foot on the ladder, will have high hopes of success and often great plans for the future. He may, in his search for success, neglect his partner and their children. This, by alienating him from his partner, may lay the foundation for sexual problems between the couple as well as for difficulties in his relationship with his children. There are many patterns to the family life of the ambitious workaholic. A typical one is that in which his wife, who has had to manage on her own most of the time, learns to be self-reliant and to reduce her need for him. Similarly, the children, used to being disciplined and to fol-lowing the rules set by their mother, may resent a father who appears from time to time and who expects them to drop everything and to do things his way. Sadly, the ambitious father often tries to justify his behaviour by telling his family and the world that he is doing it for them; that they should be grateful. He is clearly doing it for himself, but no one can refute his assertion that in material ways his family is better off than it otherwise would be.

One of the difficulties in sexual counselling is to persuade a man that he needs to spend time on his personal and sexual relationships before any problem can be resolved.

Work for a woman may be important in the early years, particularly if she is pursuing a career, but provided that she can plan her family by the use of effective contraception, she may willingly decide to temporarily abandon her career in order to have children.

Generally it is accepted that women will continue to work after marriage before having children, and indeed it is often economically necessary. This is unlikely to cause problems in the relationship other than, perhaps, a diminishing libido if a woman is expected to be responsible for, and run, the home on her own as well as go out to work. This reduction in libido may be the result of tiredness or may also be due to resentment of a situation where her partner is unwilling to share the work in the house.

Sexual Relationships

Early Stages

At some stage of a relationship, the couple will probably decide to express their feelings for each other in a sexual way and have intercourse. Whether or not the sexual relationship is able to develop without problems will depend on the upbringing of each partner, their past sexual experiences and the situation in which they find themselves. If the couple have privacy and time then the sexual as well as the general relationship will have an opportunity to develop at its own pace.

However, when each partner lives at home and parents are firmly against premarital sex, then the opportunity for sexual activity will be limited. The relationship tends to be restricted, and a rather false situation is created. Both partners may have space and time to themselves to get ready to go out, and will usually look their best. They may meet mainly in the company of other people and often with alcohol as a regular component of their meeting. They may then think that they get on well together, which is not always confirmed when they do get married or live together.

As far as the sexual relationship is concerned, this restricted meeting may have one of two main effects. It may be for the girl, if her confidence in her sexuality is not very well developed, that the lack of time and privacy will affect her sexual arousal. If she is pressured to have intercourse, say in the back of a car, she may soon become disenchanted with the whole idea of sex.

As far as the man is concerned, if there is the opportunity to have intercourse perhaps only once every two weeks, then he will feel pressured to perform adequately, to 'get it right' on this one occasion. Failure then means that by the next occasion the fear of failure is much greater – producing yet more failure. If intercourse is attempted in situations where time is restricted then even if failure of erection does not occur, it is quite likely that the boy will ejaculate quickly – thus setting the pattern for sexual functioning in the future.

The other, perhaps more common, reaction to restricted meetings is that the excitement of dressing up to go out, the alcohol, the risk of being found out having a sexual relationship will trigger a sexual response that is linked to excitement, danger, and a feeling that sex is naughty or a rebellion. Contraception will probably be used in the same haphazard way as in adolescence.

The frustrations and difficulties with lack of time and privacy may well lead to the couple living together or to marriage.

Living Together

If the couple decide to set up home together there will be the initial excitement of planning and settling in – without, however, the formalities and traditions which surround marriage. There may or may not be parental approval, which may or may not matter, often depending how close emotionally or geographically the couple are to their parents. The sexual relationship, if it has been satisfactory before, is likely to continue to be satisfactory and will develop along with the whole relationship.

However, problems arise when the relationship up to now has been fraught with difficulties of time and privacy. The couple who were unable to function sexually in these conditions may find, when living together, that they are now able to respond. On the other hand, the couple may find that the anxieties and resentments which occurred in the past continue into the living together relationship, and that the sexual relationship does not improve. The couple are likely to blame the fact that they are not married and will often tell each other that the problem will get better after they are married.

In the ordinariness of daily living, two quite separate ideas of domesticity come together and for the first time in their lives the unwashed meets the unshaven. Under these circumstances, the girl, who has functioned well sexually when the relationship was special, with an exciting or 'naughty' background and often with alcohol around, may quickly find that her libido is diminished or disappears completely.

Marriage

There are still those couples who restrict the full expression of their sexual relationship until they are married. This may be for religious reasons or because of strong moral taboos. This does not always cause problems, particularly if both partners are agreed on this course of action.

However, problems may arise. Some couples, in the premarital stage, regularly touch each other sexually – commonly called petting – until a high degree of arousal is reached and then stop abruptly because of guilt at what they are doing. This may produce a behaviour pattern which is difficult to break after marriage. The fact that full intercourse is no longer wrong, indeed is expected in the marital relationship, is not, unfortunately, always sufficient to break the previous pattern of stopping the sexual response. This can be very much to the distress of both partners.

If petting has taken place premaritally regularly to orgasm by masturbation or oral sex, with satisfaction being achieved by both partners, then when intercourse is 'allowed' after marriage it often proves to be a great disappointment. Some couples, however, use this form of love-making premaritally as a form of contraception.

Another problem may be discovered after marriage, if no pre-marital intercourse has taken place, and that is an inability to consummate the marriage – no penetration of the woman by the man is possible. This may be for several reasons; the woman may be frightened of penetration and involuntarily squeeze tight the entrance to her vagina – called 'vaginismus'; or the man may be fearful of penetrating the woman and lose his erection – called 'impotence'. Often these two conditions occur together, with the sexually fearful couple choosing each other – each recognising that the other is not a threat sexually. Before marriage they convince each other that they want to wait until marriage to have intercourse. After marriage they may try, give up, and run away from their failure either by ignoring the sexual relationship completely or by developing a satisfying sexual relationship by masturbating each other. It is often only when the couple decide that they want children that the non-consumation becomes a problem and the couple seek help.

For couples who have had premarital intercourse, similar problems may arise to those presenting when the couple decide to live together. Couples, who have convinced each other that the problem would get better on marriage, are often in for an unpleasant surprise. The greater security of marriage may allow the privacy and time for the sexual relationship to develop, but unfortunately the rituals and traditions of marriage and the myths perpetuated by the media (particularly advertising) encourage couples to believe that all will be well once they have walked down the aisle in a cloud of white lace. It then becomes very difficult for the couple to admit to themselves that they are not following this magic norm and living 'happily ever after', and even more difficult to admit it to anyone else.

Another difficulty arises with marriage – that of role stereotyping. Although this is not strictly to do with sexual functioning, the resentments that may arise because of this may well affect their sexual relationship. Role stereotyping does not seem to happen so often when the couple are living together as there are few established rules or rituals for living together – apart from perhaps in subcultures where it is the norm for a whole group of people. However, on marriage, the man becomes a 'husband' and the woman a 'wife'. Imperceptibly people tend to adopt the role that they see as appropriate to those titles. They will have developed the idea of how the 'husband' and 'wife' are expected to behave from their own parents. If the husband's parents have very different roles from the wife's parents then this may lead to great confusion in the couple as the wife acts out her mother's role and the husband acts out that of his father.

The couple may use their married friends as role models, which may or may not fit what they actually want. They may use role models from books, films or television series.

This drive to adopt roles seems to be very strong; many couples tell me how, after years of living together, their relationship changed on marriage, and seemed to take on a life of its own. A couple need a great deal of confidence and some of them may need some professional help before making the marriage *their* marriage and not that of anyone else. The importance of conforming was brought home very forcibly to me by a married couple who asked for advice about whether or not they were normal. It transpired that they were the only married couple in a block of flats – all the other couples were living together, unmarried!

Confusion and conflict may arise after marriage when the role of 'husband' conflicts with the man's previous role as 'one of the boys'. He may be subjected to ridicule by his previous 'mates' and described as 'hen-pecked' if he no longer wishes to spend the same amount of time with them. Indeed, in an attempt to assert his independence and control his fear of being swallowed up by his wife and marriage, he may continue to try to be 'one of the boys'.

Women may have similar problems, but probably less so. A woman's role conflict is more likely to be between that of her job, if she continues working, and that of a 'wife' – particularly if she sees the wife as someone who should stay at home and darn socks, do housework and cook meals.

Contraception

I do not propose to discuss here the mechanics of the various methods of contraception, merely to describe how requests for various contraceptive methods may be influenced by attitudes to sexuality or may hide pleas for help for sexual problems. Requests for changes in contraception may also be a disguise for sexual problems.

Contraception itself may be difficult for some people to reconcile with a sexual life. A common reason for this is religion. The only method of contraception acceptable to the Roman Catholic church is that of abstinence during the likely time of conception. This is not to say that Roman Catholics do not use other methods of contraception, but, if they go to confession, they have to negotiate a way of being accepted in this by the priest to whom they confess.

Muslims are generally unwilling to use contraception until they have several boy children, and not always even when they have. Boys enhance the economic status of the parents and the social standing of their mother as they bring their wives to live in their parents' home and their wives then become subordinate to their mother. Most Muslim families will go on attempting to have boy children even though there may be medical reasons for contraception.

Cultural traditions may affect attitudes to contraception. In some cultures a woman cannot prepare food if she is menstruating and so methods such as IUDs, which may prolong the period or the mini pill which may give irregular bleeding, will not be acceptable. In some cultures a woman's right hand must be kept clean, and if a diaphragm is chosen as a method of contraception, cap fitting must be taught using the left hand only.

Another reason for difficulties in reconciling contraception and a sexual life is that for some people fertility and the need for intercourse are very bound up together. Such people, and in particular, women, may lose interest in sex if there is not some chance of becoming pregnant. Consequently, the combined pill, which gives almost 100 per cent effective contraception, may be a very poor method for them, leading to pill 'forgetting' – rather like playing Russian roulette. For these women female sterilisation as a permanent method of contraception is nearly always a disaster as far as a sexual life is concerned and often leads to a request for reversal. The menopause is a particularly difficult time for the woman who sees fertility and sexual activity closely linked.

A man who has been told that he has a nil or very low sperm count may become impotent, as may a man who has had a vasectomy without realising how important is the concept of his fertility to his sexual functioning.

As previously mentioned in the section on adolescent sexuality, using contraception means accepting that one is going to have a sexual relationship, and for some people that may be difficult.

The Sheath

The sheath (condom, rubber, french letter, or sometimes just 'contraceptives') may be disliked by men, who find that their sensations during intercourse are dulled. On the other hand, men with premature ejaculation may find that they obtain a better degree of control using a sheath. The change in method of contraception from sheath to, say, the pill or vasectomy, may be sufficient for the man to experience a loss of control over his ejaculation.

Women who dislike mess and the sticky feel of semen after intercourse may find intercourse acceptable only if it is somehow sanitised with its product parcelled up in a sheath. If her partner is happy to use a sheath then this will not present a problem. Only if it is not acceptable to the man will the woman need help to come to terms with what lies behind this feeling of unacceptability of the mess.

Nurses in family planning clinics frequently come across attitudes to contraception that may suggest that the patient has difficulty in accepting some aspect of her sexuality. However, unless the patient presents with a problem, or requests help, however obscurely, it is not appropriate for the nurse to show that she thinks that the patient has a problem. One of my particular sayings in sex therapy is: 'A problem is not a problem until it is a problem!' The issue must be seen from the point of view of the patient, rather than from that of the nurse who might feel that she would certainly have a problem if she felt in the same way as the patient. Another area of difficulty with the sheath is that it must be put on the erect penis before penetration takes place. Consequently, it is intrusive and can stop the natural flow of sexual activity and may restrict the foreplay. (In some cases though, the putting on of the sheath is an enjoyable part of the foreplay.) The sheath may even cause failure of erection in some men. However, many couples do use the sheath quite happily and successfully. In fact, nearly as many couples use the sheath for their contraceptive method as use the pill.

The Cap

For a woman to use the cap (diaphragm, Dutch cap) successfully, she must have come to terms with her sexuality in a way that is not such an essential part of other contraceptive methods. Not only does inserting the cap need to be premeditated – although not necessarily just before intercourse as the cap can be inserted at any time and even worn most of the time provided that the spermicide, which must be used as well, is inserted just before intercourse takes place – it needs the ability to touch the genitals, to insert something into the vagina and to add to the wetness that will be created by semen by inserting a cream, jelly or foam spermicide. The insertion of spermicidal pessaries which are made of cream in solid form, is less messy and obtrusive, but these have to melt to be effective and then they add to the amount of stickiness after intercourse.

Provided that the woman can cope with this, the use of the cap gives a great deal of freedom and autonomy in contraception without interfering with her body in any way.

One example of a request for a change in contraception not being quite what it appeared to be, was when a patient, whose partner had used the sheath, apparently successfully, for many years, requested a change to the cap. On the face of it it appeared to be a straightforward request for a method change but it was important for the nurse to understand why the change was being requested and what were the patient's expectations of the new method. On questioning, the patient stated that yes, her husband was happy with the sheath. When she was asked what it was about the cap that she thought would suit her better, she replied with a question, checking her understanding that she would have to use a spermicide with the cap. What turned out to be her problem was one of dryness on intercourse, which she thought the spermicide would help to overcome. It was important to check that this did not mask a cry for help about a more deep-seated sexual problem, but in this case, it did not seem to do so. In fact, it was revealed that both or them preferred to use a sheath and the addition of either a spermicidal jelly or lubricating jelly was what was required, rather than a change of contraceptive method.

When fitting a cap and teaching the woman to insert and remove it herself, fears and fantasies are often revealed about the size and shape of the vagina. An opportunity should be given to the patient to express these fears and time should be taken to educate as necessary.

The Combined Pill

There is a great deal of controversy about whether or not the pill causes a loss of interest in sex. Statistically, apparently, there is no proof of this. However, it may be that some patients, perhaps because of the freedom from anxiety about pregnancy, have an increased libido on the pill. These patients would numerically cancel out the patients who have a decreased libido.

Admittedly, it is easy to blame the pill for a loss in libido when it may be that there are factors in the relationship which are affecting sexual response; even worry about being on the pill may cause excuses to be found to blame the pill. Nevertheless, I am convinced that certain pills – notably those containing 0.25 mg levo-norgestrol – do have, for certain women, an adverse effect on the libido. If these women are changed to a different pill, containing a different and less powerful progestogen, then often their libido returns, without any other therapy.

A request for the pill may mask difficulties that a woman has with her sexuality, as putting something in one's mouth, at a time unconnected with intercourse, is very different from, say, inserting a cap. However, unless the patient gives some hint or clue that there is a problem, it would be quite unreasonable to suspect the millions of women who do take the pill of sexual problems. The pill is a highly effective, convenient method of contraception for those for whom it is suitable.

Sterilisation

Requests for sterilisation often mask an underlying sexual or marital problem. A couple may have tried all the other methods of contraception, blaming each in turn for the problem. They may then feel that if they are sterilised, with freedom from worry about pregnancy, then all will be well. Unfortunately, all may not be well, and indeed the sterilisation may add to their problem, particularly if the partner who has been sterilised has been persuaded to have the operation by the promise that it will change everything. The ensuing resentment, if it is found that the problem has not been resolved, is likely to make the problem worse.

It is important for people being sterilised to answer the question, 'How would I feel being *sterile*?' and, if their partner were to die, or they were to separate, 'Can I enter into another relationship knowing that I cannot have children of that relationship?' Too often a couple take the decision as to which of them should be sterilised, based on information about how easy the operation is for either of them. I really feel that this is one of the least important issues. The difference, in any case, is only measured in days, unless there are medical problems, whereas the result lasts for many years. The psychological effects for a man may be greater than for a woman, as his fertility could have been expected to continue for the rest of his life. A woman's fertility is already acknowledged as ending at the menopause and she may thus find the further shortening of her span of fertility easier to cope with. Reversal is possible in some cases, but it is not the best idea to think in terms of a possible reversal when contemplating sterilisation. Patients who have not thought through this concept of sterility are the ones likely to have sexual problems following sterilisation.

Infertility

As previously mentioned, fertility, for some people, is very bound up with their sexual functioning. Unfortunately, society expects a couple to produce children, even if they are not very inclined to do so. Pressure from parents and in-laws may start soon after marriage, and friends who one by one become pregnant lead the couple to ask

'What is wrong with us?'

Again, unfortunately, people commonly are ignorant of what is the normal time that it takes to become pregnant. The chance of pregnancy on any one act of intercourse is only 3 per cent (Tietze, 1960) rising to 30 per cent just before ovulation (Barrett *et al*, 1969). Most couples, if asked, would say that three to six months is the time that, after which, if they are not pregnant, then there is something wrong. Fertility varies from couple to couple, and decreases with age. It may be perfectly normal for someone aged 30 to take two years to become pregnant. It is also important that patients understand the time of the month that conception is likely.

The effort of trying to become pregnant, keeping temperature charts, going to the hospital for tests and having intercourse on the 'right' day can put a great deal of strain on a couple's sexual relationship. While actively trying to become pregnant, the woman's libido may remain high, only to fall when she does become pregnant or is told that there is no hope. The man may become impotent because of having to produce an erection to order. These stresses will place the relationship under strain – which in turn will affect sexual functioning.

There may be a chemical factor working as well. The hormone prolactin, produced by the anterior pituitary gland, is raised in stress, and prolactin may inhibit both ovulation and sexual drive, thus compounding the problem.

One possibility that the nurse must be aware of is that the patient presenting with infertility may have come for quite another reason. A couple who have been unable to consummate their marriage are often reluctant to seek help, as it means admitting their failure. One way that they may choose to ask for help is by going to a family planning clinic, or their GP, for advice on infertility. They see it as more acceptable to say that they cannot become pregnant than that they cannot have intercourse. It is important when seeing a couple requesting advice for infertility, to check with them that they are in fact having vaginal intercourse.

Pregnancy and Childbirth

Sexual problems may arise during pregnancy, but it is unusual for patients to seek help at that time, as the problem is often seen as a temporary one, attributable to pregnancy.

Questions are often asked during pregnancy about the advisability of having intercourse. As the uterine contractions associated with orgasm may be sufficient to induce premature labour (Goodlin, 1969), care should be taken if premature labour is threatened. Other contraindications for intercourse are bleeding in *this* pregnancy, an incompetent cervix, pre-eclampsia or ruptured membranes. However, apart from these conditions, no harm can come from intercourse during pregnancy. Indeed, intercourse at full term, because of the prostaglandins in the semen, may be a very successful way to induce labour. This may be suggested to women as an alternative to an induction of labour. An unnecessary ban on intercourse at this time may well lead to sexual problems later. It may be necessary to change the position used for intercourse – for example, to one where the couple lie on their sides with the man entering the woman from behind. Couples should be encouraged to find a position, however unusual, which suits them.

Either partner may decide to abstain from intercourse because of fear of harming the baby, either by the thrusting, or by introducing infection. Sometimes the semen is seen as potentially 'dirty' and therefore harmful. A nurse needs to be aware of likely fears and counter them with education during pregnancy (Glover, 1983). Nurses should be aware that a woman who does not enjoy intercourse may attempt to manipulate them, or the doctor, into banning intercourse so that she can tell her husband that she has been told they must abstain. If this situation arises it must be identified and discussed with the patient, who may be using this approach to ask for help with her sexual problem.

Sexual problems following the birth of a child can often be traced back to events surrounding pregnancy.

Role Change

If a woman becomes pregnant before she embarks on a career, or before the couple have come to rely on two salaries, then becoming pregnant may not significantly change the woman's role – particularly if the woman is happy to see herself as a mother. However, for a career woman, the change of role and activity is very marked and may lead to the woman becoming very unsure of herself in her new role. The role of 'mother' may conflict with her role as 'wife' or 'sexual person', particularly if she has been programmed to believe that 'mothers' don't have sex.

In addition, the gestational age of the fetus is not related to the emotional 'gestation' of the mother – some mothers become very conscious of their child and relate to it quickly, and others hardly relate to it at all. In the middle the majority have days of enjoying being a prospective 'mum' and days of dread and confusion which they are frightened to admit. The nurse needs to help the woman to understand how she is feeling and to educate her partner so that he will support her.

Change of Body Image

Some women revel in the idea of pregnancy, their skin becomes clear and luminous and their hair glossy. They feel successful, happy and healthy, once the early morning sickness has been over-come, and see their change in shape as a kind of badge of office. However, others find this altered shape very difficult to accept. They see themselves as big, fat and unattractive; they worry about stretch marks and drooping breasts following breast feeding; they feel thoroughly asexual. Their partner may have similar reactions – either pride in his wife's appearance or disgust at what he may see as her obscene shape.

Parental Support

Women may vary in their acceptance of support from their parents. For some it is a relief to know that their mother has been through the experience and will be on hand to cope. For others, however, the thought of their mothers intruding, taking over, is very fright-ening, and they will feel they must do it 'their way' in order to retain their identity.

Parents will also differ in their acceptance of their impending role as grandparents. For some it will be a pleasant anticipation, and bring back happy memories; others may feel angry, feeling they are being called upon to participate in something in which they had no choice, fearing that their freedom may be curtailed once the baby arrives.

Fears

A woman may have fears that she cannot cope with motherhood; fears of pregnancy and childbirth; apprehension about induction of labour, episiotomy, stitches and admission to hospital; dislike of the necessary gynaecological examinations and the lack of privacy and the waiting for ante-natal care.

Childbirth and Afterwards

Problems related to the delivery of the baby such as prolonged labour, forceps, episiotomy and stitches or emergency caesarian section, may all affect a woman's attitude to her sexuality. A woman who has adverse experiences during pregnancy, childbirth and afterwards will come to associate sexual activity with these unpleasant experiences and may avoid intercourse in the future in case it leads to pregnancy and a repetition of the experiences. Even women on the pill and therefore relatively safe from pregnancy may still feel an underlying distaste for sex – related to experiences surrounding childbirth.

Breast feeding, sometimes a struggle, sometimes extremely pleasurable, can distance a mother from her partner. She may feel that her breasts, once a source of pleasure for herself and her partner, should be kept for her child. Indeed, she may get some degree of sexual satisfaction from breast feeding. However, her partner may feel very pushed out particularly as the woman's breasts may be tender from feeding and so she may be unwilling to have her partner touch them. In addition to this, the raised prolactin levels associated with breast feeding may depress her sexual desire.

The effort of breast feeding however, may be just one of the many things which tire the new mother. Not the least of these is the need to be on duty, as it were, for 24 hours a day, with total responsibility and little sleep. Small wonder that it affects her sexuality.

Another aspect of having the baby, is the effect the baby has on sexual activity between the couple, by being in the same room as them at night. This seems to worry women more than men. Even though it is obvious that the baby can have no idea about the sexual activity of its parents, many women find it very inhibiting, almost as if their parents were in the same room.

Childbirth itself – involving as it does the stretching of the vagina, which plays a major part in a woman's lubrication system, and the stretching of the entry to the vagina with possibly bruising and stitches – can cause, from the physiological point of view, difficulties in regaining sexual functioning. The length of time required for a woman to be ready for intercourse after childbirth seems to vary enormously. Some women seem to be looking forward to intercourse almost immediately, while others will not be ready until at least three months after delivery. The nurse can help the woman in the post-natal period to understand why she has a lowered libido.

If the woman does not feel ready for intercourse by the time of her post-natal examination, she can be encouraged to have sexual activity with her partner other than intercourse. The use of a lubricating jelly is very helpful after stitches.

Equally, however, the nurse may need to give permission for the woman to resume intercourse well before her post-natal, advising, of course, on the use of contraception. Provided that a woman feels sexually aroused, then she is ready for intercourse.

Unwanted Pregnancy

I have called this section 'unwanted' rather than 'unplanned' pregnancy, because often, once the question of pregnancy has been established, and after initial doubts, the couple will look forward with pleasure to the birth of an unplanned child. Indeed, as previously mentioned, it is this spice of a possible pregnancy that is an integral part of sexual enjoyment for some couples, and for women in particular.

Unwanted pregnancy may occur to married and unmarried couples as well as to women when single or as a result of an extra-marital affair. When the pregnancy occurs within a marital relationship, it is not often seen by outsiders as a tragedy. However, if the pregnancy continues, it may well create unacceptable financial burdens for the couple. These burdens will then affect the marital relationship and probably the sexual relationship.

The degree of resentment felt about the pregnancy may depend to some extent on whose 'fault' it appears to be. A wife who 'forgot' the pill, may be accused of manipulating the situation so that she can have the baby that her husband has declared they cannot afford (and indeed she may have done just that). The husband who refused to use the sheath, which was their previously agreed method of contraception, and who has a wife who finds the thought of coping with any more children completely abhorrent, may find that his wife's future sexuality is destroyed by a burning resentment.

Other disagreements between the couple about contraception may often lead to an unwanted pregnancy. However, contraceptive method failures, such as a sheath bursting, are less likely to affect the relationship, as there is something to blame other than themselves.

Unmarried couples living together may find that the unwanted pregnancy upsets the balance of their relationship. Sometimes there may be the suspicion that one partner has laid a trap for the other so as to force him or her into a marriage, as couples often do decide to marry when expecting a child.

Unwanted pregnancy, for the single girl, particularly if she is young, will produce many pressures from society and from parents. The latter may tend to use phrases such as 'Scandal', 'What will the neighbours say?', 'How could you let us down?' – with emphasis on their feelings rather than their daughter's feelings. Conflicting messages may be given by her peers, who may feel that the pregnancy is rather exciting and a declaration of independence. Either way, the girl is likely to feel confused and guilty.

A girl who has actively tried to become pregnant in the hope of trapping her boyfriend may find that the pregnancy is not so wanted after all, when faced with the anger of her parents and the desertion of her boyfriend. Fears about being found out, may lead the girl with an unwanted pregnancy to consciously conceal the pregnancy from her parents and friends. She may conceal the fact from herself by refusing to acknowledge that her periods have stopped and that she is getting bigger.

Unwanted pregnancy for the married woman having an extra-marital affair, may be dealt with by her making sure that she is having intercourse with her husband as well, so that it will be relatively easy to pass off the baby as his. A problem has arisen with the increasing number of men who have had vasectomies and who then have to blame the surgeon for what is in fact infidelity on the part of the man's wife. Problems also arise if the extra-marital partner is of another race. Confrontations after the birth of the baby are not uncommon.

In this group of women, provided that the marital relationship is reasonably satisfactory, the sexuality of either partner is not likely to be affected. However, if the affair is indicative of underlying difficulties, then a pregnancy may signal the end of the sexual relationship – either because the woman no longer wishes to have sex with her husband, or because the man cannot live with the treachery of his wife once he has found out.

For each of the other groups of women, the unwanted pregnancy is likely to affect their future sexuality by associating sex with something unpleasant, and thus making them want to avoid a possible recurrence of the unpleasantness – and so they avoid sex if possible.

Abortion

In the previous section, the question of the unwanted pregnancy was discussed as if the pregnancy was to continue. However, for many people abortion is seen as an alternative.

As far as the mortality of the operation is concerned, abortion in the first trimester is much safer than pregnancy and childbirth, than the pill taken by smokers of all ages and by non-smokers over the age of 30. Abortion is only just less safe than the pill for non-smokers up to the age of 30 (Tietze *et al.*, 1979). However, from the medical point of view there are associated problems of infection, possibly leading to a blocked tube.

As far as the effect on the woman, research has shown that from the psychological point of view the effects of abortion are not as great as the effects of continuing with an unwanted pregnancy (Brewer, 1977). The crucial factors seem to be the degree of guilt about the abortion and whether the woman has been able to grieve for the child. The former may depend on the woman's religious upbringing and the attitude of her parents both in her childhood and about the abortion. The latter is influenced by being surrounded by people, particularly parents, who insist that the girl has the abortion and then urge her to forget all about it. Somehow it becomes as if it had never happened. I have found many instances of loss of or lack of libido in women who have had an abortion and who have never had the chance to talk about how they felt about being pregnant or about having the abortion. . Grief often manifests itself on the anniversary of the abortion or the expected birth date of the aborted child.

The woman may have felt pressurised by her partner into making a decision to have an abortion. A form of blackmail may have been used, with the partner threatening to leave if the woman refuses to consider abortion. Such pressures may lead to resentment which will affect future sexual functioning. However, sometimes men are not consulted by their partners, and become angry as they would have liked to have a child.

Nevertheless, I do believe that if a woman has had an opportunity to share her feelings about the pregnancy, has been allowed a real choice as to whether or not to continue with the pregnancy or to have an abortion, and to discuss how she feels afterwards, the chances of the abortion affecting her future sexuality are very low.

Nurses have an important role to play in this field, not only in formal abortion counselling, but as community or clinic nurses when the pregnancy is confirmed, and in the gynaecology ward where the abortion takes place. Here staff attitudes to abortion can be crucial for the sexual health of the woman. If following the termination the woman is depressed, or unable to come to terms with what has taken place, she should be advised to seek help from her general practitioner or health visitor.

Still-birth

I would like to make a plea here for the needs of the mother to be understood when she has a dead baby. Fortunately, the attitudes which were common in the past that 'The least said, soonest mended' and advice to 'Go home dear and have another baby as soon as possible' are being superseded by those showing a greater understanding and sensitivity.

After a still-birth, the mother, and father as well, not surprisingly are upset. Often the father, in order to cope with his own grief, colludes with the staff to shelter the mother from what they see as a greater upset, and so does not encourage her to see the baby. However, if she is not allowed to see and hold the baby, it is likely to remain a fantasy thing – not taken into the reality of her own experience. It will never die.

A mother of a stillborn baby needs to cry, to mourn the baby that has been such a vital part of her emotionally as well as physically, for the past months. It may be that seeing and touching the baby is necessary for the healing process to begin.

Nurses may feel that they have failed if they are unable to give the mother the baby for which she has waited nine months, and this may affect how they deal with the mother. Suggesting that she goes home as soon as possible may be their way of dealing with the feelings that are difficult to cope with. If the nurse is able to recognise and come to terms with her own feelings of grief and failure, then she is more likely to be able to help the parents. One practice that is being introduced is that of taking a photograph of the baby. If the parents refuse the initial offer, the photograph could be kept in the notes in case the parents change their minds later.

One patient came to see me complaining of loss of libido, several years after the birth of a stillborn baby. She had not seen the baby or had anything to do with the disposal of its body. A friend told her that they burned still-births in the hospital incinerator. It was not until I traced the birth and found where it was buried in a local cemetary, so that they could go and mourn, that she was able to face a sexual life again.

13   40–60 YEARS: MIDDLE LIFE

As in the chapter on the period 20–40 years, the life events which occur during the time from 40–60 years, will be discussed, together with their effects on sexuality.

Work

Work for a man and for a woman, during these years, will, in general, have different meanings.

Some men will have been promoted, perhaps many times, and often, in the course of these promotions, will have been working away from home and losing contact with their wives and families. Having got to the top of their particular trees, they may now be looking for different sorts of satisfactions, perhaps feeling vaguely uneasy at the lack of satisfaction in their success.

Some men in this situation may look for a relationship outside marriage, which in itself may add to their feelings of dissastis-faction. Even though the man could function adequately, sexually, with his wife, he may find that he is unable to obtain or maintain an erection with this new sexual partner – because of anxiety that he will not come up to scratch, or be seen as old and past it by a younger woman.

Other men, to combat this lack of satisfaction at their success, may seek a closer relationship with their wives and families. This approach may be welcomed, but is just as likely to be rejected. Wives who have been left on their own to manage, often resentful at the neglect, have, nevertheless, often managed to cope successfully, building up in the process a life which relies on satisfactions other than those provided (or not) by their partner. These are not neces-sarily sexual satisfactions, but may be from children, friends, work or other outside activities. The reappearance of their husbands, wanting a closer relationship, may well stir up old resentments and create new ones, as their wives find the time that they are giving to the other activities questioned by their husbands. This new situation may well produce sexual problems in either partner and they will often need help to re-adjust.

Instead of obtaining promotion, a man who had high hopes of achievement at work in his twenties and thirties may well in his forties and fifties have to face up to the reality that he is not going to get anywhere. Men who have not had the preoccupation of bringing up a family in the earlier years, and for whom work has been very important, may find disillusionment setting in; a feeling of failure; of having nowhere to go.

There does not seem to be an identifiable hormonal change in these years as there is with women, but there does seem to be what is described as a midlife crisis for men, a feeling of being past 40 or past 50, when they seem to lose their sense of purpose. This disillusionment may affect his sexual functioning, and as described with the high fliers, may lead to frantic affairs with younger women to try to regain the feeling of power and potency – both sexually and in his general life. It may also lead to his rediscovering girlie magazines in an attempt to stimulate his fading desire, or it may lead to apathy in his sex life – to a giving up. A single episode of sexual failure at this time may be the start of total impotence.

Fears of unemployment, of redundancy, of being passed over for a younger man all affect the self-esteem and often the potency of men. Pressures of work, physical, mental and emotional, also have their effect on a man's sexual drive. These can occur at any age, but perhaps more so as a man gets older, together with perhaps an expectancy of a naturally occurring diminishing sex drive and performance.

For women, work at this time of life may be much more exciting. A woman who has given up her career to have children may be beginning to look around, now that the children are older, to see how she can resume her career. She may be thinking of a new career, as the opportunities for retraining are now, generally, greater than they were. She may find that this new life outside the home gives her a new-found energy and sense of purpose. This may be reflected in a new surge of sexual energy which will not always fit in with her partner's perhaps depressed sexual drive. It may be that these new activities provide opportunities for meeting a new sexual partner, which may then be threatening to her marital relationship.

The Menopause (Climacteric)

This seems to be an exclusively female phenomenon, with no real counterpart in men. The term 'menopause' means, simply, the cessation of periods, and occurs on average around the age of 50 years. The word 'climacteric' is used to describe the whole range of changes which characterise this time, and which may spread over a period from 40 to 60 years (Bancroft, 1983).

There are three main effects of the climacteric on a woman's sexuality.

Loss of Oestrogen

This causes a change in the lining of the vagina with a resultant loss in the ability to lubricate. Consequently, the vagina may become dry and sore. As with many other 'normal' phenomena, an explanation to the patient may be all that is required, together with advice on the use of lubricating jelly. However, if the symptoms persist, oestrogen-containing creams are very effective. Alternatively, the woman may need hormone replacement therapy if she has many debilitating symptoms; this will also improve the atropic vagina.

Loss of Fertility

As mentioned earlier, for some women, sexuality is very bound up with fertility. The realisation that their fertile life has now ended may cause these women to refuse to continue with a sexual relationship.

Unfortunately, the climacteric often occurs at the same time as children are leaving home, thus ending her life as a mother. She may react to this double sense of loss by turning away from her partner, or by becoming more demanding, expecting him now to supply the emotional satisfaction that she received from her children previously. The emotional and possibly sexual pressures may have disastrous effects on her partner's potency.

Change in Mood

At the climacteric, chemical changes take place in the brain as a result of changing hormone levels, and these may alter the moods of women. This feeling of not being in control of herself, of feeling a different person, may have a marked effect on the woman's sexuality.

However, care should be taken that all changes in mood are not ascribed to lack of oestrogen. Glandular activity generally is in an altered state and thyroid dysfunction and diabetes may occur, masked by other symptoms of the menopause. A thorough medical examination should be encouraged.

In the same way that the two previous stages of 20–40 years and 40–60 years had characteristic role changes, the 60+ stage has its own particular characteristics.

Men, in particular, may find it very difficult to adapt to the idea of retirement. The lifestyle of the last 40 years changes abruptly, the sense of purpose, of worth, may disappear overnight, and adjustment to retirement may involve a type of grieving.

For a woman, a different adjustment may need to be made, particularly if she has never worked, or has retired earlier than her partner. Now, instead of planning her day, on her own, doing exactly as she wishes, she has her partner at home as well, maybe interfering and criticising what she is doing (possibly in an attempt to make some purpose for his own empty life).

How the two of them work out this period of change will affect how they relate to each other sexually. It is necessary for mental and physical health, for each person to develop his life in a way that is as satisfying as possible; for each to maintain some privacy and individuality and not to become totally dependant on the other. This way, there is a good chance that the emotional and sexual life of the couple will improve.

Sexual Functioning

People generally expect the incidence of sexual activity to fall with age – indeed there seems to be an expectation by the young that old people do not have sexual relationships. Relationships, particularly sexual ones, between old people are often derided by their families who see it as somehow threatening and 'not very nice'. It is impossible to judge how much of this is in order to cover up fears of the financial implications of a bereaved parent marrying again and leaving his wealth to his new wife rather than just living alone till death and leaving his wealth to his family. Nevertheless, the idea of sex between two people aged 70 years seems to make younger people uneasy.

There is no evidence that women lose their sexual drive or enjoy sex any less as they get older, apart from problems directly related to low oestrogen levels of the climacteric. Their sexual activity may be less, but that may be because, as men die at a younger age than women, there are less men around with whom to have a sexual relationship.

As far as men are concerned, the general view was that men's sexual interest waned in later life, but most studies have taken a cross-section of the population at different ages and measured sexual activity. Any differences here might reflect different attitudes to sex at different ages rather than how the sexual functioning of particular individuals changed. However, a longitudinal study (George and Weiller, 1981) showed that men who had an active sexual life, particularly if they started at an early age, continued unimpaired throughout old age.

As far as change in performance is concerned, there is a tendency for less frequent early morning erections, a longer time and more stimulation needed to obtain a full erection, less warning of impending ejaculation, a reduced volume of ejaculate, and a longer refractory period.

With increasing age, the chances of illness are greater, with its corresponding effect on sexual functioning. Also a period of abstinence from intercourse may give difficulties in restarting.

Physically Handicapped

One of the greatest difficulties of the physically handicapped, concerning their sexuality, is that they are generally considered by others to be asexual. Because their bodies are often distorted, or their speech impaired, it is beyond many people's imagination to believe that handicapped people are capable of wanting and achieving a sexual life. Not only are the physically handicapped deprived of an identity – the 'Does he take sugar in his tea' attitude – they are often treated as children, and thus sexual activity is seen as inappropriate.

Handicapped children are less likely to receive sex education than other children, which makes entering adulthood more difficult, and, because they may need their parents to continue to provide intimate care, they will find it difficult to make the separation from their parents, which is a prerequisite of adult sexuality.

Greengross (1976) suggests that society has an underlying fear that handicapped people will reproduce, producing a baby even more grotesque than themselves, which will ultimately undermine and weaken society. Parents also have a fear of their child's becoming pregnant, so that they would then have to cope with yet another child. Parents also tend to monitor their children's relationships, desperately hoping that someone will come along who will look after their child when they are dead. Unfortunately, this hope is likely to be unrealistic, and in the process denies the child the opportunity to make caring relationships, however transient or imperfect (Greengross, 1976).

Reality for the handicapped is that, although they may feel inside their outer shell that they are 'normal', with hopes, fears and feelings similar to those of the non-handicapped, they are unable to act out or express them. Similarly, in sexual relationships they may have identical sexual needs and responses to the non-handicapped, but be unable, because of their disability, to achieve the full range of sexual activities that are possible for the non-handicapped.

The nurse who is involved in caring for the handicapped may need to give basic sex education, including emotional as well as sexual aspects, to encourage them to go out and to make relationships as much as is possible, and may need to give permission for them to be sexual, and to discuss contraception if intercourse is likely to be possible. She should also be sensitive to their need for privacy. She may need to be imaginative, suggesting possible ways to overcome the physical disability in order that the person may make some kind of sexual contact – not necessarily intercourse. Aids such as vibrators may be necessary to help someone masturbate, if his fingers cannot reach, or do not work effectively.

It is beyond the scope of this book to list the disabilities and ways of coping sexually, but there is an organisation, Sexual Problems of the Disabled (SPOD), which produces very useful literature and is happy to respond to requests for help and advice.

Mentally Handicapped

Mentally handicapped people may also be physically handicapped, with all the same difficulties. On the other hand, they may be very physically attractive, with a childlike quality which may add to their attractiveness. This may create even greater fears in their parents, or others responsible for caring for them.

Fears of pregnancy, of exploitation, are legitimate fears, but there are other fears that are unlikely to be acknowleged. Mentally handicapped people often have a lack of awareness of society's constraints on the open display of sexuality. This lack of inhibition may cause unease in the carers, who themselves may not have come to terms with their own sexuality, thus causing them to be restrictive about the sexual expression of their charges, in order to protect themselves. There is often a double standard regarding the sexual activities of the mentally handicapped, with a stricter standard of sexual behaviour and morals expected of them than would be expected of non-handicapped people.

There are probably even greater fears about mentally handicapped people reproducing than there are about the physically handicapped. Greengross (1976) reviews the surveys of fertility and stability of relationships in the mentally handicapped, and concludes that these fears are unfounded – partly because of lowered fertility levels, and partly because sexual expression is more likely to be in the area of kissing and cuddling, and sleeping together, than sexual intercourse.

Sex education needs to be given to each mentally handicapped person, individually tailored to his limit of understanding. They also need education about what behaviour is acceptable in public and what, such as masturbation, should be carried out in private. The question of contraception needs to be carefully considered, with, as for anyone not handicapped, an assessment made as to the method which is best for that person.

Suggested Further Reading for Part III

Delvin, David, *The Book of Love* (New English Library, 1974).
Greengross, Wendy, *Entitled to Love* (National Marriage Guidance Council, 1976).
Stewart, W., *The Sexual Side of Handicap* (Woodhead Falkner, 1979).
Zilbergeld, B., *Men and Sex* (Fontana, 1978).

PART IV

SEXUAL PROBLEMS

The preceding parts of the book dealt with the development of sexuality and how that sexuality fitted into a person's life. This part of the book will deal with the difficulties and dissatisfactions that people have with their sexual life.

Whether a person sees his dissatisfaction with his sexual life as a sexual 'problem', to be treated or cured, may depend on his understanding of what is normal, or on his expectations of the relationship. In other words, two people may be in an identical situation, as far as their sexual functioning is concerned, and yet one may see the situation as a 'problem' and the other as 'That's the way of life'.

People may also differ in what they see as the causes of their sexual problems. It may be seen entirely as a medical problem, in which case they may seek help from a doctor; as a marital problem, in which case they may try another relationship or seek help from a marriage guidance counsellor; they may even see it as something to do with their lifestyle, in which case they may try to move house. If they are correct in their assessment of the cause of their difficulties, their choice of solution may lead to the resolution of the problem.

Frequently, though, patients are mistaken in their assessment of the cause of their problem and the nurse's role, if she is the one to whom they turn, is to help them to sort out what is the cause of the problem, so that they may be appropriately referred.

In order to do this, the nurse needs to understand the terms commonly used in dealing with sexual problems and something about each type of problem.

Lack of Libido

Other terms for this are total unresponsiveness, inhibited sexual desire or frigidity. This means someone who has never experienced sexual desire or arousal, and therefore has probably never been orgasmic. Almost certainly, the cause is to be found in the way that the person's sexuality has developed in childhood – either because of punitive actions by parents towards the manifestations of sexuality in childhood (such as masturbation), incest or rape in childhood; or it may have a physiological cause in that the sexual and reproductive system has not developed adequately.

Loss of Libido

This is secondary unresponsiveness or frigidity – a lack of sexual desire, or arousal in someone who has previously been responsive.
   Some of the common causes:–

Physical
— after childbirth
— after repeated vaginal infections, eg, monilia
— after repeated cystitis
— after previous pain on intercourse
— dry vagina at the menopause
— drugs
— the 'pill'
— hormone inbalance

Emotional
— tiredness, eg, from caring for small children
— presence of a baby in the room
— fears of harming the baby in pregnancy
— marital disharmony
— no longer seeing the partner as a sexual partner
— parents or in-laws in the next room

111

— only wanting sex in order to have a child
— poor body image
— following hysterectomy, mastectomy or colostomy
— depression

Anorgasmia

This means failure to achieve orgasm. It may present as the person
never having had an orgasm, failing to have an orgasm on intercourse without manual stimulation, or failure of orgasm after
having previously been orgasmic.

Common causes
— failure to lead up to intercourse and to stimulate the clitoris
  adequately
— inability (associated with anxiety, fear, and so on), to allow the
  orgasm to happen
— anger towards the partner causing withholding of the orgasm
— pattern set up pre-maritally of petting leading to 'cut off' when
  guilt became too great
— fear of sexual response due to incident in childhood – also
  leading to 'cut off'
— fear of being out of control in a woman with a controlling
  personality

Vaginismus

This is a spasm of the muscles surrounding the outer third of the
vagina, preventing penetration by the penis (and in many cases by
anything else). This usually occurs as a primary condition, and once
it has been treated it rarely recurs. However, it may develop as a
secondary condition in someone who has experienced a particularly
difficult birth, or other traumatic experience, such as rape.

The cause of vaginismus may be very difficult to establish in any
particular case. Sometimes it is possible to identify incidents in the
person's past which could account for it; usually though, it is completely inexplicable. Luckily, it is not necessary to discover the
cause in order to treat it. Often the women are very attractive, and
respond quite normally, sexually, even having regular orgasms

manually, as part of an active sex life apart from intercourse. Thus treating the vaginismus is very rewarding, as once the phobia of having the penis in the vagina is overcome, the couple's relationship usually blossoms quite remarkably.

However, some cases of vaginismus are part of a general sexual unresponsiveness, when the whole sexuality is depressed. These patients are far more difficult to treat, as they seem to have many deep-seated problems. It is commonly discovered when women refuse a vaginal examination, or respond badly to an examination.

By and large, male sexual dysfunction mirrors female dysfunction – which is not surprising as the physiology is basically similar.

Erectile Problems Or Impotence

The two words frigidity and impotence have come to mean much more than just failure of sexual functioning; they are used as a description of personality, so that the labels 'frigid' and 'impotent' carry with them a whole host of negative attributes. Consequently, the term erectile problems more accurately describes what is meant here – which is failure of erection. This may be *primary*, arising from difficulties of sexual development – either physical or emotional. Other distinctions may be made between total failure of erection, failure to penetrate or between failure in any situation or failure only with some people or in some situations.

Secondary erectile failure arises in someone who has previously functioned successfully.

Physical causes

— diabetes – 50 per cent of sufferers have difficulty
— drugs – hypotensives, tranquillisers
— alcohol
— nerve damage in trauma or disease
— hormonal inbalance
— other medical conditions (see 'Physical Causes'. p.117)

Emotional causes

— worries about job
— overbearing or belittling women
— performance anxiety following one episode of failure
— new relationship after previous relationship ended
— infertility
— depression

Premature Ejaculation

Definitions vary as to what constitutes premature ejaculation. However, I consider it to be ejaculation before entry, or within a few thrusts of the penis after entry, and without any sense of control.

This is a condition which has no female counterpart, as an early orgasm in a woman is usually no problem, as she could go on to have further orgasms. A man, though, because of the refractory period, is unable to achieve another erection immediately.

Premature ejaculation may be seen as a failure of learning to control a body function, in the same way that control is gained over urinating or defaecating. A common history is of frequent masturbation, or intercourse in hurried circumstances. It *may* be connected with anger in the relationship – used as a subconscious means of thwarting his partner's pleasure.

However, a man who has been without sexual relief for some time will almost always ejaculate quickly the next time he attempts intercourse.

Failure to Ejaculate

Or retarded ejaculation – which is the counterpart of anorgasmia. This may be divided into two types: *Retrograde* ejaculation, which is ejaculation and orgasm, but with the semen entering the bladder – as may happen in diabetes or after prostatectomy. *Failure* to ejaculate, which is often linked with men who need to keep tight control of themselves. Alcohol is a frequent cause of failure to ejaculate as it dulls the sensations and thus adequate stimulation cannot be achieved. Drugs may also affect the ability to ejaculate. Patients suffering from spinal injuries or multiple sclerosis may find difficulty ejaculating even if they achieve erection.

Joint Dysfunctions

A type of primary erectile difficulty may occur in the partner of a woman who experiences vaginismus. While she has this problem, the man will have no difficulty maintaining his erection, merely not attempting intercourse too actively, saying that he does not want to hurt her. However, as the treatment of his partner progresses, he will show reluctance to co-operate with instructions about 'homework', and when she is able to accept penetration, he will develop erectile failure.

It is important to recognise this as a joint dysfunction – often brought about by an immature man marrying an immature woman, their relationship being quite satisfactory, with sex pushed into the background. However, once they decide to have children, the balance changes, creating problems. The man is usually content to see his wife as the one with the problem, but when she is treated, he has to face up to his own difficulties. It is essential that they are treated together.

At other times the partner presenting with the problem is not the partner with the main problem. One common pair of conditions is that of the woman who presents with loss of libido, but on taking the sexual history it is found that her partner has always suffered from premature ejaculation, thus causing a woman with normal libido to lose interest in sex after repeatedly failing to be sexually satisfied.

Another joint problem is the man presenting with erectile difficulties whose partner, because of her lack of libido, quietly sabotages his attempts, by verbal and non-verbal cues to show that she does not want him, and yet can triumphantly tell him that it is all his fault.

It has been the trend for those treating patients with sexual problems to assume that these problems were largely psychological in origin. Initially, problems were seen in psychoanalytic terms as being the result of some deep-seated emotional conflict which manifested itself as a sexual problem in order to protect the psyche from further conflict. Masters and Johnson (1970) introduced the idea of seeing sexual problems in behavioural terms, as faulty learning or as conditions arising from the stimulus-response phenomenon where a painful or unpleasant episode occurred at the same time as sex – thus linking the two and causing problems in the future.

Many therapists, notably Kaplan (1974), see problems as a mixture of the two. However, in many cases the cause may be found to be relatively simple – faulty understanding or an unhelpful situation in which the couple find themselves.

One area which has been ignored until recently is that of physical causes, even though patients often tend to see their problem in those terms. Rather than assume that the cause is psychological, it makes sense to exclude physical causes before any form of therapy is undertaken.

The causes of sexual problems will be discussed in terms of the physical, the individual, the relationship, the educational and situational.

Physical Causes

Age

The effects of ageing are often difficult to assess, nevertheless there does seem to be a general trend of the slowing of sensitivity and reactions – particularly in men in the lengthening of their refractory period and time taken to achieve an erection. However, when adopting an 'It's never too late, policy with older patients, I have seen some dramatic changes in sexual functioning; not necessarily back to the vigour of their youth, but a vastly improved satisfaction in their sexual relationship, with, often, a realisation that sexual pleasure may be given and received in ways other than vaginal intercourse.

General Illness

Any illness, at any age, will affect sexual functioning. If a person is preoccupied with how awful he is feeling, then it is unlikely that his libido will be very high. The 'headache' is the classic excuse, but it may in fact be a reality. The chronic tiredness of the mother with young children really fits into this category. Chronic illness has an even greater effect on sexuality, leading often to introspection and a change in roles between partners – from relating as man and woman to becoming as parent and child.

Heart Disease

After a heart attack, advice is usually given regarding the amount of exercise a patient should take; however, specific discussion about future sexual activity is often missed out. Because of this, patients feel uncertain as to how it will affect them. Even if they are given advice, and this must depend on the medical condition of the individual patient, it may go unheard, and the fear often remains that they will have another heart attack and die during intercourse. Even if the patient does not have this fear, his partner may fear this and thus find that it destroys her ability to enjoy sex. Bancroft (1983) suggests that intercourse within a stable relationship is beneficial after a heart attack, but that the stress of intercourse during an extra-marital affair is more likely to lead to problems. Angina during intercourse may be countered by taking coronary dilators before intercourse, or by modifying positions in order to lessen the amount of effort.

Arteriosclerosis and Cardiac Failure. These may affect sexual functioning, particularly in men, and that these conditions may result in poor blood flow to the penis and thus lead to erectile difficulties. These conditions probably affect women less, as they do not need such an efficient blood supply for their sexual performance and the neurological effects of clitoral stimulation are unimpaired. Digoxin, commonly given for heart failure, also seems to have an adverse effect on sexual functioning.

Hypertension

This may cause difficulty in two respects; it may be associated with arteriosclerosis as above, or its treatment with Beta blocking drugs will almost certainly give rise to impaired sexual functioning.

Renal Failure

The incidence of sexual problems in patients with chronic renal failure is very high (Kolodny *et al.*, 1979) as well as the incidence of amenorrhoea and reduced fertility. There may be several reasons – changed hormone and other blood chemical levels, change in blood flow to the genitals and, almost certainly, the general debilitating effect of chronic illness.

Diabetes

Around 50 per cent of males with diabetes have erectile problems (Wagner and Green, 1981) and it is often the presenting problem in young male diabetics. Thus urine tests for sugar, followed by blood tests if suspicious, are essential for men presenting with erectile problems.

This disease is another example of a chronic illness causing sexual problems as well as neurological and vascular pathology which becomes worse with increasing age. Problems seem to be related to peripheral neuropathy rather than retinopathy (Wagner, 1981) and are of an insidious onset. Retrograde ejaculation is a common feature.

However, although 50 per cent of diabetic males have sexual problems, 50 per cent do not. As there is no way of distinguishing for certain which patients have a physical cause, treatment should be geared to the assumption that the patient is one of the 50 per cent not affected. Women seem to be much less affected sexually by diabetes, although there is a higher incidence of monilia which may affect sexual functioning.

Multiple Sclerosis

This is another condition in which sexual problems are common. They are often linked to urinary problems – in that similar nerves are affected. However, the fact that the patient may have a catheter will also affect sexual functioning. Many patients do not realise that it is possible for men to strap the catheter alongside the penis in order to penetrate, or for the woman to attach the catheter to her abdomen, thus keeping it out of the way during intercourse. Fear of urinating during intercourse may be helped by passing urine before commencing. Adductor spasms in women may be particularly distressing and make intercourse difficult.

The lack of a sweating reflex in the pelvis and lower limbs has been linked with the incidence of sexual problems (Wagner and Green, 1981). However, as in diabetes, doctors sometimes automatically attribute a patient's sexual problems to his multiple sclerosis. I have found it unhelpful automatically to assume that they are connected, and feel that each case should be investigated and a careful sexual history taken.

Spinal Cord Injuries

People tend to think that patients with spinal injuries are unable to function sexually. However, unless the sacral section of the cord is destroyed, a man may have reflex erections even though the central appreciation of the feeling is not the same as before. Similarly, he may be 'turned on' from the sex centres in the hypothalamus if the lesion is below T8 (Higgins, 1979).

Consequently, it is possible for both men and women to continue to have intercourse once they have recovered from the initial trauma. They will still have an orgasm, but it is likely to feel different, possibly less intense, than before the injury. What is more likely to happen is that erection is possible, but that ejaculation is impaired, as the amount of stimulation needed after the injury may be greater than before, and certainly greater than provided on intercourse. The use of vibrator as an alternative or adjunct to intercourse may help in this case.

Another feature of spinal injuries is that touching the body, above the injury, may assume a greater erotic significance as if to make up for the deficiency below. (Kolodny *et al.*, 1979).

Epilepsy

A rather confused picture emerges regarding the effect of epilepsy on sexual problems. There are links between temporal lobe epilepsy and sexual variations such as fetishism and transvestism, but as young epileptics are likely to have a disturbed childhood, it is impossible to separate out this component. In addition, drugs used for epilepsy are suspected of having a depressing effect on sexual drive, possibly by altering hormonal levels (Bancroft, 1983).

Ileostomy and Colostomy

Because of the possibility of damage to nerves supplying the genital area occurring in these operations, which usually involve extensive surgery, it is quite likely that sexual functioning will be affected subsequently. However, even if that were not so, the altered body image caused by having a smelly, unpredictable opening in the abdomen, covered by a plastic bag, must be sufficient to make someone have second thoughts about wanting to expose his body in a sexual relationship.

Patients with ostomies need careful counselling and support, and may find an organisation such as the Ileostomy Association helpful. Other disfiguring operations such as *mastectomy* and *vulvectomy* may have a similar effect on body image and self-esteem.

Prostatectomy

This may lead to two types of problem. Some degree of retrograde or 'dry' ejaculation is common in all types of prostatectomy, because of the damage to the internal sphincter of the bladder. However, after the more extensive perineal prostatectomy, usually for carinoma of the bladder, erectile problems are likely to occur because of damage to the nerve supply. Again, it is important that patients are given a clear understanding of what has been done to them, and reassurance given that in most cases, it will not affect sexual functioning, apart from retrograde ejaculation.

Genital Abnormalities

There are several relatively uncommon conditions of the penis which will affect sexual functioning.

Priapism, which is a long-standing erection, classed as a surgical emergency, may lead to erectile difficulties in the future. *Peyronies Disease* consists of fibrous plaques in the penis causing deformity of the erect penis, so that it bends downwards in the middle, which is both embarrassing and painful. *Hypospadis* is a congenital abornamilty where the opening of the urethra is on the underside of the penis, causing problems with erection and ejaculation. *Phimosis* is inflammation of a too tight foreskin.

In women, lack of lubrication at the menopause, repeated monilial or other vaginal infections or episiotomy or badly sewn tears following childbirth, may all cause problems on intercourse. A rigid hymen may prevent entry and inflamed Bartholins cysts may cause pain on intercourse. Pain on deep thrusting of the penis may be caused by a retroverted uterus or pelvic inflammatory disease.

Endocrine Disorders

The effect of hormones on sexuality is very complex. Androgens are

linked to sexual desire in both sexes; however, the level of circula-
ting testosterone is not an adequate test on its own, as the amount of
free testosterone depends on Serum Hormone Binding Globulin
(SHBG). It is the amount of free testosterone which affects sexual
drive. Increased prolactin and an imbalance of T_3 and T_4 will depress
drive. A complete hormonal assay of T_3, T_4 FSH, tesosterone,
SHBG and prolactin, together with blood sugar, is necessary to
exclude problems associated with hormonal effects.

The combined contraceptive pill is, of course, a hormone. Studies
on the effect of this on sexual drive are conflicting (Bancroft, 1983).
Nevertheless, I believe that women presenting with loss of libido on
the pill, should first have the progestogen content of the pill reduced
and changed, and then, if possible, have two or three pill-free
months before being treated further for their sexual problem –
unless, of course, it is clear from their history that the problem is
unconnected with the pill.

Psychiatric Disorders

The main psychiatric disorder to be linked with sexual problems is
endogenous depression. Loss of libido is an early sign in depression
and one of the last symptoms to be resolved. This may be because of
a general lack of feelings of well being, which seem necessary for
sexual drive, but also because of the chemical changes in the brain
which take place in depression. Unfortunately, drugs given to treat
the condition may also cause problems – in particular, monoamine
oxidase inhibitors commonly lead to ejaculatory failure (Bancroft,
1983).

Other psychiatric disorders such as *mania* or *hypomania* may
increase sexual drive, but not necessarily sexual functioning.

Impairment of sexual desire and performance has been linked to
most of the psychotropic drugs, but it is extremely difficult to
separate effects due to the psychiatric condition.

Alcohol

It was generally thought that, in small amounts, alcohol increased
the libido by reducing central control. However, Wilson and
Lawson (1976) found in experiments that the effect of small
amounts of alcohol was related to learned expectations of the effect
of alcohol rather than to the chemical effect. Consequently, it is
possible that any increased libido is an expected effect of alcohol,
rather than an actual effect.

Moderate amounts of alcohol may make ejaculation difficult as it will lead to a dulling of sensation.

In larger amounts, alcohol frequently causes sexual problems. It is difficult to separate the physical effects of the habitual use of large amounts of alcohol, from the effects of the alcohol on the relationship. Also, it is possible that an acute alcoholic episode will produce erectile failure, which in itself will produce fear of failure subsequently, and thus start a vicious circle.

Long-term effects of alcohol may produce peripheral neuropathy and endocrine changes – but it is not clear whether they themselves result in sexual difficulties. There has been a suggestion that Disulfram (Antabuse) is responsible for erectile or ejaculatory problems, but this is not substantiated by other studies (Wagner and Green, 1981).

Problems in the Individual

In a sexual relationship, a person brings to that relationship himself, as a person, as well as his body. Consequently, the way he functions and relates as an individual will affect how he functions and relates sexually. In a sexual relationship, a person's defences are down, he is open to both physical and emotional attack and therefore he needs to be able to allow himself to be vulnerable, to have learned to trust another person.

In the part of this book that dealt with the development of sexuality in childhood, the various stages of development were discussed. Difficulties at any of these stages may affect how a person relates to another, sexually, and also the attitude of the parents to sex over the whole of the person's childhood will influence how he develops as a sexual person.

Repressive Childhood

In the most extreme cases of repression in childhood not only is anything to do with sex seen as wrong, but any activity that is seen as the child taking the initiative and developing his own personality, will be frowned upon and discouraged. This may lead to the adult being frightened to enter into a relationship with someone else, for fear of rejection and punishment. Punishment at the time of sexual exploration may lead to anxiety being experienced whenever sexual feelings are aroused in the future.

Religious ideas may also add weight to the feeling that sex, and in particular masturbation, is wrong. By the time marriage is contemplated, the taboos are often too strong to break.

Feelings of Disgust

These feelings may be connected with feelings about other body functions, particularly defaecating. The wetness of lubrication or of semen may be seen as messy and distasteful by either partner, and great attention to hygiene may be shown. The person will often be fastidious about body smells, and about the smell of semen in particular.

The person may well have had over-scrupulous parents, who themselves could not tolerate mess. These feelings of disgust may show themselves as a phobia of the genitals, either of their own, or of their partners.

The sheath is likely to be the preferred method of contraception.

Self Control

The aspect of sex over which the individual has no control, once it has started, is orgasm. Thus orgasm may be difficult for people who are anxious about losing control. This anxiety may be connected with masturbation as an adolescent and fears that they will be unable to control themselves once they start, and will become addicted.

A woman may fear that she will come to like sex too much and become promiscuous. She may settle for an unexciting partner with whom she has no fear of losing control. People who fear the rising excitement of sexual arousal, may rush towards penetration before they are properly aroused and then complain that they cannot achieve orgasm. They subconsciously see the sensuous foreplay as a threat and tend not to like this part of lovemaking.

Fear of Injury

Psychoanalytic theory abounds with explanations of sexual problems in terms of fears of castration, penis envy, and incest taboos resulting from Oedipal conflicts. These explanations are difficult to prove or disprove, but patients do express fears of damage to their penis or their vagina – of being ripped open, lost inside the abdomen through an open-ended vagina, of abdominal contents falling out if the labia are parted, and of the penis being 'bitten off' by the vagina.

Fears are also expressed by the patient that he will cause damage to his partner rather than being damaged himself.

Sometimes, of course, the fear of injury is real and related to past assault.

Vulnerability to Stress

Kaplan (1974) suggests that, as some people under stress develop gastric ulcers, headaches, or hypertension, others develop problems of sexual functioning in situations in which other people, without this vulnerability, would not. This is not quite the same thing as people who fear failure – which may itself cause anxiety, and thus compound the failure. Others, however, may fear success, and will start to sabotage their treatment once they begin to improve.

Spectatoring

This is described as a person watching himself to see how his sexual responses are progressing. It is particularly counter-productive to achieving orgasm, as the essential here is to 'lie back' and let it happen.

However, too much detachment is as bad. Looking at the ceiling and counting the cobwebs, or planning tomorrow's shopping or car repairs, is not conducive to good sexual performance. A certain amount of focusing on the pleasure being experienced is also essential.

Personality

It has been suggested that certain personality types are linked with the occurrence of sexual problems, but no real evidence has emerged (Bancroft, 1983). Nevertheless, of the people who do develop sexual problems, those that have obsessive, perfectionist traits, seem to have great difficulty in carrying out non-demanding pleasuring exercises, which are meant to take away the pressure of performance and to allow sexual arousal to occur spontaneously. The perfectionist finds it difficult to tolerate the fact that his penis will not rise to order, and insists on turning the pleasuring exercises into an activity which he has to perform correctly and in being perfectionist about the exercises destroys their object – that of helping him to relax and cease performing.

People who have outgoing personalities may well be able to mask the fact that they have problems, as they need to be seen as confident and competent. It may take some practice before the nurse is able to recognise the vulnerability beneath the veneer of cheerfulness.

Self-esteem

A person with poor self-esteem, with feelings of inferiority, will generally find difficulty in establishing a sexual relationship. These feelings of low self-esteem may be linked to depression (which will need treating) or to body image, particularly in connection with mutilating surgery. Far less obvious aspects of body image may also affect self-esteem – too large or too small breasts, thick or thin legs, general body shape, size of penis, may all affect how a person thinks of himself as a sexual person.

Need to Please the Partner

The need to please one's partner, rather than take sexual pleasure for oneself, is basically a failure on the part of a person to see himself as 'good enough' – with rights to pleasure of his own. Instead, he needs to be 'good', placating, and may feel that his partner will become angry if her needs are not satisfied. Consequently, the woman may struggle to have an orgasm that she does not really want, in order that her partner may feel that he can give her one. Continually being preoccupied with the sexual pleasure of her partner may spoil her own pleasure – for example, she may feel that 'If I take too long to come, he will get tired' and thus in effect delay her orgasm.

Underlying this, also, is often a failure of communication between the couple, with one partner unable to ask the other to touch him or her in a way that is particularly pleasurable. Women often find difficulty with this, as there seem to be more taboos about women enjoying sex. If it happens by accident, as it were, then that seems to be all right; however, women generally find it difficult, or shameful, to ask for sexual pleasure. They may resent the fact that an accident of this kind is not repeated, and lie there willing it to happen, but without offering a clue.

Problems in the Relationship

It is not necessary to have a deep and lasting relationship in order to have a sexual relationship which is physically satisfying. Sexual attraction between two people may arise quickly, followed by sexual arousal and satisfaction, leading to a feeling of well being and pleasure, provided that the experience is entered into freely by both partners.

However, before becoming fully satisfactory for both partners, sexual activity between two people may need some practice and thus it is unlikely that the satisfactions arising from the 'one-off' sexual experience will be as rewarding as those experienced as a relationship develops. A sexual relationship may become increasingly an important way of expressing the closeness and sharing in the relationship and may then become a source of emotional as well as physical satisfaction. When a sexual relationship is part of a close emotional relationship, then factors in that relationship are likely to affect sexual functioning. When faced with patients complaining of sexual problems, it is essential to establish the part that the relationship plays in their sexual functioning.

No Commitment

Quite commonly, when seeing a couple complaining that one of the partners has 'gone off sex' it is rather difficult when seeing them together, to establish a cause. However, if the partners are seen individually, it may be revealed that one partner has no commitment to the relationship – either because he is contemplating leaving, or because he has another relationship. Either way, he is often reluctant to reveal this to his partner. In these circumstances, it is unrealistic to treat the loss of libido.

No Seuxal Attraction

Another cause of lack of interest in sex is when one partner does not see the other as a sexual partner. Two people may establish a relationship for reasons of status, economy, security or companionship. They are not necessarily sexually attracted to one another. One example of this is when a homosexual marries in order to prove, either to himself or to others, that he is heterosexual. The relationship may be a disaster sexually, if he is unable to find his partner sexually desirable.

A relationship which did include sexual attraction at one stage, may, because of a change in the physical appearance or personal habits of one of the partners, become an asexual relationship on the part of the other partner. This may be because of weight gain or loss, smoking, alcohol, mutilating surgery, or because of a deliberate attempt on the part of one uninterested partner to appear sexually unattractive – he is then able to blame their sexual problems on the partner's lack of interest.

Unresponsive Partner

A person who initially has a normal libido with adequate sexual functioning may present with loss of libido. It may then be found that his partner has, because of her own sexual problems, developed subtle ways of 'turning him off' – such as described above. There are other ways – such as sighing, loudly, whenever a tentative hand is stretched out; making sure that he is asleep in bed whenever she comes upstairs; staying up to watch late TV or video until the partner gives up and goes to bed; insisting that the dog/cat/baby sleeps between them; headache; backache; tiredness; continual menstrual period; these are all ways that may be used to 'turn off' a partner – who eventually stops trying and in self-defence becomes asexual.

Belittling Partner

The unresponsive partner displays a passive form of anti-sexual behaviour – the belittling partner is far more active. Seeking to achieve the same result, a woman may complain about the size of a man's penis and compare it unfavourably with others she has known. On being asked if she enjoyed a sexual episode, she may reply, 'Oh! Have you started?' or, just as he is becoming excited, 'Haven't you finished yet?'

A man may continually run down his partner's appearance – particularly her breasts or legs, features which she is unable to alter. Either partner may chatter incessantly, laugh at the wrong moment, or constantly accuse the other of being less of a person; of failing them; of being no good. It is very difficult for anyone, however adequate sexually, to maintain that adequacy in the face of such belittling.

Overdemanding Partner

When there is a great disparity of sexual need between partners, then problems are likely to occur. What seems to happen is that as one partner pressures the other, the other actually wants sex less. This sets up a vicious spiral; as one moves towards the other, the other moves away, thus making the first partner attempt to get even closer. In the end, the pursuing partner is likely to be asking for sex more often than he really wants in the desperate hope that 'tonight he may be lucky!'

The couple need help to see how their behaviour is making the problem worse; and that if one backs off a little, then this will give the other a chance to move towards them, rather than running away.

Role Expectations

When two people form a relationship, each brings to that relationship a set of expectations as to how the other will behave. These expectations arise partly from how their respective parents behaved towards each other, how the relationships of friends were structured, and partly from previous relationships. If both partners have had similar experiences, then all will be well, but if they come from different backgrounds, perhaps even different races or cultures, then problems may be expected.

These differences may be made worse if communication between the couple is poor. Resentments may build up over something as mundane as whose job it is to clean the windows, make early-morning tea, or tend the garden.

A woman whose father always took her mother a cup of tea in bed before leaving for work may feel very unloved by a man who tiptoes out of the bedroom when he leaves early for work, yet his idea of caring may be to leave his partner undisturbed.

If assumptions such as these are made without checking them with each other, then problems in the relationship may soon appear.

Other aspects of role expectations may cause difficulty. A man who has a traditional view of marriage may feel that marriage entitles him, in return for the financial upkeep of his wife, to sex, meals, housekeeping and childbearing. A wife who does not have the same expectations, may feel that sex if something that should be shared when they both feel like it. Her husband may feel very affronted at not being able to exercise his marital 'rights' whenever he chooses.

Unresolved Conflicts

Resentment between partners is a very frequent cause of sexual problems. Battles conducted outside the sexual relationship often spill over into that side of the relationship, with one partner withholding sexual responsiveness in order to get back at the other.

'He needn't think he is going to win all the time.' 'If he won't be nice to me, then I'm not going to be nice to him.' 'If she is going to shout at me every time I do something she doesn't like, I shan't bother to try (sexually).' These sentiments are often expressed by clients. The effect on their sexual functioning may be conscious and deliberate, or subconscious and come as a surprise to them when the connection between their feelings and their lack of sexual response is pointed out.

One common area of difficulty is money, or lack of it. Couples frequently have different expectations of how to spend money – again this is often related to their different backgrounds, and may emphasise the woman's dependence on the man when she is unable to work during motherhood.

Another area is work. Who will go out to work; for how much; may the wife earn more than her husband; hours of work; weekend work – all these have potential for conflict. A woman may feel undervalued as a housewife, particularly if the man stresses how often she is able to sit down during the day and plan her own time. A man may feel his work is undervalued when his wife accuses him of working only eight hours while she works for twenty-four hours – with maybe a job as well as the responsibility for the home.

Children are a frequent cause of resentment between a couple, particularly as they are often adept at coming between parents – given the chance. Again, each partner will have his own ideas about bringing up the children. Discipline, pocket-money, the degree and type of involvement of each partner, schooling, and choice of friends – these are all areas for potential conflict.

Communication

The inability to communicate one's needs, and feelings of joy pleasure, fear and anger, to one's partner, is, I believe, at the root of many sexual problems. The difficulties discussed in the two previous sections, role expectations and unresolved conflicts, flourish when either partner is afraid or unable to express his needs and feelings clearly.

Often a person will not understand what is happening. He will experience anger, perhaps at something his partner has done, or even from an incident at work. He will then react, acting out his anger, perhaps by refusing to speak or by replying 'Nothing' when asked what is the matter. If he is more active he may react by slamming doors or shouting at the children.

His partner, in response to this inexplicable show of unpleasantness, may react by withdrawing, or retaliating, depending on individual style. A situation has then arisen where two people are upset, neither clearly knowing what has caused their problem. This may then carry over into their sexual relationship.

Someone who is frightened about an aspect of his life, the children or perhaps an illness, may be unable to express this fear, and keep it bottled up – affecting his behaviour in a way that is quite inexplicable to his partner. She may then feel that she is the cause of the upset, but dare not ask. A breakdown in communication then causes suffering in the relationship.

Women, in particular, seem to set up an obstacle course for their men – expecting them to know by some kind of instinct what are their emotional and sexual needs. 'If he loves me, he should *know* what I like' is frequently expressed. Often the woman is afraid to acknowledge her sexual needs, and feels that to ask for sexual pleasure is cheap, dirty or degrading. If the man happens by accident on what she likes, then all is well. If not, then she may lie silently fuming, feeling that he is useless, and thus destroying her sexual responses in the process.

The first step in helping people to communicate is to get them to acknowledge their needs and to recognise their feelings. The second step is to teach them to express verbally the needs or feelings, rather than to act them out. If they can be helped to realise that each person is responsible for the satisfaction of his own needs, rather than his partner being responsible, then they can learn to help their partner help them.

Communication difficulties may cause sexual problems by causing difficulties in the relationship, which then extend to the sexual relationship. However, communication difficulties may exacerbate existing sexual problems, making it even more difficult to resolve them.

A man who has a failure of erection on one occasion, may become tense on a subsequent occasion, fearing further failure – thus causing that which he feared. His anger with himself may cause him to be brusque with his partner, who may then feel doubly rejected. Her reaction to this may compound his problem. However, an open sharing of fears and disappointments will reduce the tension and make further failure less likely.

Educational Causes

Lack of Knowledge about the Body

Despite formal sex education at school and the availability of many books on the subject, many people remain ignorant about their bodies and how they function. They piece together snippets of information gleaned in childhood and from friends, and never bother to check the accuracy of these early formed ideas.

Many women have no clear idea about their vagina, and even less idea of their clitoris. Fears and fantasies abound regarding their vagina. Probably their failure to check reality is linked to being unable fully to accept their sexuality. They seem to 'not want to know!'

Men, too, are often unsure about women's sexual organs and sexual functioning. If they are not confident about their sexuality, they may express this by not knowing where to put their penis in intercourse, or being rather fearful of causing damage, unsure of how hard to push.

If either partner is able to express these fears to a nurse, then it is relatively simple and very rewarding to give an anatomy lesson – with the woman holding a mirror and her partner looking on and both touching as appropriate. As well as demonstrating her anatomy, permission is being given to look, touch, and to accept that part of the body.

There seems to be less uncertainty about male anatomy (probably because it is more easily seen than the woman's) apart from about the size of the penis when flaccid in relation to size when erect or to performance. Occasionally, the tensing and lifting of the scrotum is seen as abnormal. More uncertainties are concerned with function, or about the composition of semen – particularly after a vasectomy. Since the sperm are a very small component of semen, explanations are often needed as to how, and from where, semen arises.

Realities of Sexual Performance

Even if people are clear about their sexual anatomy, they are often ignorant about the way that their bodies work. Despite much being written in popular magazines, both men and women still expect that the norm for women is that she will have an orgasm on intercourse alone, without any stimulation of the clitoris either before or during intercourse. On the other hand, couples may have been led by the magazines to believe that unless the woman has multiple orgasms then something is wrong. Often both partners expect that they should have an orgasm simultaneously and that is one has an orgasm, without the other doing so, then a great failure has occurred.

Men often expect to continue to achieve several erections a night and feel that the need for more manual stimulation of their penis as they get older, is a failure.

People expect to perform well sexually even when they are drunk, tired, ill, unemployed or in their parents' house.

Nurses need to have a clear idea of what it is reasonable to expect in order to help patients who complain of sexual problems to put them in perspective.

Sex Role Stereotyping

A common view of male/female roles in sexual activity is of the man as the dominant initiator, with the woman the passive receiver. If the couple share this idea and are happy with it, then all is well. However, people do have different ideas. Frequently, men feel that if they have always to initiate lovemaking, then the woman is not interested in them. Many men find that an initiating and imaginative woman is a tremendous 'turn on' and welcome her aggressiveness. Other men, however, find this threatening to their role.

In these circumstances, it is essential that the couple communicate their likes and dislikes and that the nurse emphasises that there is no right or wrong way. Each couple need to work out the balance for themselves.

Situational Causes

A couple may have no difficulties in their relationship, have uneventfully developed into sexual adults, understand their sexual functioning and indeed, have had a previously adequate sexual relationship, and yet still develop sexual problems – even if there are no physical causes.

The causes of these problems, which I have labelled 'situational', have been discussed to some extent under the heading of adult sexuality, where the effect of life events on sexuality was considered. Some of th se are restated briefly below.

Work

This is a common cause of sexual problems. Tiredness or absence from home may affect both the relationship and sexual functioning. Premature ejaculation is made worse by infrequent intercourse, and where there is pressure to perform on a particular occasion, erectile difficulties may arise. Lack of libido in either partner is common when overworking.

Unemployment or fear of redundancy is linked with self-image and so sexual performance may be affected either by decreasing libido or by increasing the requests for reassurance through intercourse.

Housing

There may be difficulties with privacy as described below, either because of others in the room, or because of thin walls. Semi-detached or terraced houses may cause problems – with fears of the neighbours hearing. I struggled for a long time to try to help one couple – the woman complained of loss of libido – with little success. However, I met her sometime afterwards and she told me that all was now well. They had moved to a well detached house and she now felt secure and unobserved.

Privacy

This is often linked with difficulties with housing. Living with in-laws may cause problems, both in terms of privacy and by reintroducing the parent/child relationship – in which sex is inappropriate for the child.

Privacy may be difficult with young children, if they are not taught that it is unacceptable to enter their parents' bedroom without knocking. Equally, the presence of older children may inhibit parents, who fear that their children will hear the noises of lovemaking. It may be helpful to put a lock on the door in the first instance, or move the bed away from the children's wall in the second.

Lack of privacy as parents is often linked with the difficulty of ensuring that time is still spent together as a couple, separate from the children.

Young adults, however, may find that lack of privacy outside the home, as well as in their parents' house, will affect their sexual relationship. Sex in a car, in a field, up a dark alley or behind the Youth Club, in an atmosphere of 'Quick, before someone sees,' is unlikely to help a young man's sexual performance, or to allow a girl's sexuality to develop.

Time

The previous point involved the importance of time as well as privacy. Lack of time may, in some instances, add a sense of urgency, which in itself is exciting, and thus raise the libido. However, the pressure of lack of time is more likely to lead to sexual difficulties. Any situation in which anxiety is raised is likely to affect sexual performance. Thus patients who present with a story of infrequent, snatched meetings, in places that are not altogether private, with very little time, need to understand that it is very common for people in such circumstances to have difficulties with their sexual functioning. Indeed, it is really not appropriate to try to treat their problem, other than to explain how their situation is causing the problem.

Another aspect of time affecting sexual function is at the start of a relationship. It is fairly unrealistic to expect that the first few times that a couple make love, it will be satisfactory. The anxieties of wanting to perform well will affect their ability to do so, and in any case it is unlikely that the partners will be able to communicate their sexual likes and dislikes straight away. It is far more common to need some period of adjustment and settling down, before mutual satisfaction is achieved.

Consequently, someone who goes from one relationship to another, in search of sexual satisfaction, is unlikely to achieve what he is seeking.

Fertility

Problems may arise from all aspects of fertility. The need for contraception interferes with the spontaneity of sex – some methods, such as the sheath, being more obtrusive than others. Fear of pregnancy may be very inhibiting to sexual relationships; on the other hand, attempting to become pregnant can have equally disastrous results.

If sexuality and fertility are very bound up together, then the completion of the family, sterilisation, the menopause, or a hysterectomy, may have a dampening effect on sexual pleasure.

All these aspects are dealt with more fully in Part III, but fertility together with work, housing, privacy, and time, are all situational causes of sexual problems.

Homosexuality

A homosexual relationship is a sexual relationship between two members of the same sex. The term 'lesbian' is usually used for female homosexuals, whereas the term 'homosexual' is often taken to refer to males.

Kinsey *et al.*, (1948) reported that 4 per cent of adult males were exclusively homosexual although the figures were revised to 3 per cent by Gagnon and Simon (1973) by removing criminal and delinquent males. They found that under 1 per cent of females were exclusively homosexual.

Homosexuality is commonly seen as deviant behaviour, the explanations of which range from its being a sin, to its being an illness. Society generally finds homosexuality very threatening, leading to tremendous pressure on homosexuals to be either punished or cured.

The background and implications of homosexuality are very complex, and I do not propose to write at length here as Bancroft (1983) reviews the subject in a very helpful way. However, there are a few main points that I would like to make about homosexuals so that nurses, who may come across patients who admit to being homosexual, are able to treat them with the same understanding that they offer to their ostensibly heterosexual patients.

As far as the physiology of sexual response is concerned, homosexuals are identical to heterosexuals. However, sexual fantasies are likely to be about the same sex rather than about the opposite sex, so that although the stimulus to the hypothalamus is the same, the source of the stimulus is different.

Homosexuals use similar methods of sexual stimulation as heterosexuals – such as body touching, touching the penis or clitoris, insertion of objects into the vagina in the case of lesbians or anal intercourse in the case of male homosexuals. (This latter variation of the sexual act is also used by heterosexuals, for whom it is always illegal, even between husband and wife. However, anal intercourse is legal between consenting homosexuals over the age of 21 years.)

136

Most of the stereotypes associated with homosexuals are untrue or restricted to a minority. Examples of common stereotypes are: the identifying of homosexual couples in terms of the heterosexual stereotype of male and female, with females being 'queens'; lesbians are similarly divided into 'butch' and 'femme'; that male homosexuals are effeminate in gesture and speech.

Some examples of these stereotypes undoubtedly exist, but it is likely that they will be the most obvious and therefore noticed. There may, of course, be other facets of their personality that they are expressing in their need to be noticed – not necessarily connected with their homosexuality.

Homosexuals have the same need as heterosexuals for self-esteem, to be needed and to be in close contact with another person. The nurse's role, when confronted with a homosexual asking for help, is to offer the same understanding and support that she would offer to any patient.

Homosexuals may present with similar sexual dysfunctions to heterosexuals or they may present with role confusion, guilty at their sexual orientation. They may have been unable to accept their sexuality and have married, in an attempt to prove that they are 'normal', so that marital breakdown may be the presenting symptom. They may be attending the psychiatric department in an attempt to be 'cured'. They may be convinced that they are homosexual but because of pressures from family, work, or religion, wish that they were not so.

I believe that it is unethical for nurses to be involved in 'curing' homosexuals – the nurse's role is to offer counselling and support to enable a patient to find an identity that he can be comfortable with and can live with. The nurse should also realise that it is not only among her patients that she may have to relate to homosexuals. They are also likely to be found among colleagues, friends and family. She may even be homosexual herself.

Bisexuality

The previous discussion centred mainly on exclusively homosexual men or women. However, the reality of life is that people generally cannot be neatly labelled homosexual or heterosexual. Kinsey (1948) provided a useful way of looking at the subject, by producing the Kinsey Scale (Table 19.1). Even after being established at a point on that scale, a person may move his position on the scale. It also shows that a person may have both homosexual and heterosexual relationships at the same time.

Table 19.1: The Kinsey Scale

---

0   Exclusively heterosexual with no homosexual
1   Predominantly heterosexual, only incidental homosexual.
2   Predominantly heterosexual, but more than incidentally homosexual.
3   Equally heterosexual and homosexual.
4   Predominantly homosexual, but more than incidentally heterosexual.
5   Predominantly homosexual, but incidentally heterosexual.
6   Exclusively homosexual.

Source: A.G. Kinsey, W.B. Pomeroy, C.E. Martin, *Sexual Behaviour in the Human Male* (Saunders, Philadelphia, 1948).

It would appear that many people have had homosexual contacts. Gagnon and Simon (1973) found that 30 per cent of males had had a homosexual experience in which at least one of the partners had achieved orgasm. Often these experiences are in adolescence as part of sexual experimentation. Another common time for homosexual relationships is in single-sex schools, segregated workplaces, or in penal institutions. Under these circumstances people find that the need for a close relationship is stronger than the need for a relationship with a member of the opposite sex.

However, because of society's punitive attitude towards homosexuality, people often feel guilty about these episodes and need help to realise that they are not heading for moral destruction.

Fetishism

Particular parts of the body, articles of clothing, boots and shoes, or substances such as rubber, plastic or fur are often items which are closely connected by the fetishist with his sexual arousal.

This connection may vary from being an adjunct to, or variation in, his relationship with his partner, to being an all-consuming passion, without which he cannot function sexually, and which may totally exclude his partner.

Explanations of fetishism vary according to different theorists. Psychoanalytic theory links it clearly with a severe fear of castration (Greenacre, 1979). Behaviourists link fetishism with an association of the particular object with sexual arousal and erection of the penis.

Whatever the cause, the problem usually presents when the use of the fetish is upsetting the sexual relationship with his partner. Indeed, the partner's willingness to accept the fetish as part of their lovemaking, may be crucial to their continuing relationship. Exhortations to the one to 'give it up' or to the other 'to learn to live with it' are unlikely to work. Often long-term counselling may be needed. There may be no solution.

Transvestism and Transexuality

A transvestite, or cross-dresser, is one who wears clothes of the opposite sex, either in private or in public.

In males, this need to cross-dress may be a type of fetish in which the clothes are used as a sexual stimulus and an aid to masturbation.

Another aspect of transvestism, is that, in donning the clothes of the opposite sex, the person assumes, albeit temporarily, the identity of the opposite sex. A male transvestite may feel that there is a feminine side to his personality which can only be expressed when he is dressed as a woman. Thus his masculinity is expressed in a sexual way with his partner, when he is dressed (or undressed) as a man, and his femininity is expressed in an asexual way when he is dressed as a woman. He is heterosexually orientated, rather than homosexual.

Provided that he can manage to keep both sides of his life separate, and that his partner can accept this, then this may continue in a stable state for many years. Help will be needed if the transvestism affects the relationship or if guilt at the cross-dressing is overwhelming.

However, Bancroft (1983) considers that in many cases there is a shift from transvestite to transexual. Here the person loses his original gender identity and permanently assumes the identity of the opposite sex – believing that he should really be that sex and that he is in the wrong body.

Bancroft (1983) also sees this an an attempt to reconcile the homosexuality of the person by becoming the opposite sex – which then allows an approved heterosexual relationship.

In order to have the surgical intervention needed to change sex, the person is often required to live as a member of the opposite sex for at least eighteen months in order to adapt to the proposed role. It also necessitates undergoing extensive hormonal therapy, clinical assessment and counselling. It is important that the sex change operation is not seen as a solution to all the person's problems; indeed it may create others, as the person will not be seen, legally, as a member of the opposite sex, neither will he be able to marry in his new identity.

The previous section described sexual minorities and dealt with behaviour which neither involved using force, nor was generally exploiting. There are laws which govern minority behaviour, as there are for all sexual behaviour, but these are usually concerned with preventing one person from indulging in sexual activity with another against the will (or at an age below which he is not considered able to give consent).

However, some types of sexual activity are always considered to be an offence – such as exhibitionism, paedophilia, incest and rape.

Exhibitionism

The majority of men convicted for indecent exposure are over 21 (Rooth, 1972), although the trend seems to be for a sharp increase in adolescents aged 17 to 21 being convicted.

As with all sexual minority behaviour it is difficult to classify people into types, or to conjecture about causes. However, the general pattern seems to be of immature men who find it difficult to make sexual relationships with women, or who resort to this behaviour at times of stress.

Exhibitionists tend to be young looking, and mainly approach pre-pubertal girls. The exposure is sometimes of an erect penis and may involve masturbation, whereas in other people there does not seem to be a sexual component of the exposure. What does seem clear is that the exhibitionist needs the victim to be shocked or disgusted.

It would appear to be a common experience for women – Gittleson *et al.* (1978) found that 44 per cent of a group of nurses had experienced a man exposing himself, with, however, little residual effect on them. Understanding, and help to become more 'assertive' in their relationships with women, are what the nurse may be able to contribute to the patient's development, so that he can be helped not to need this behaviour in order to assert himself.

Paedophilia

Paedophiles, like exhibitionists, may be seen as men (usually) who are unable to sustain a sexual relationship with a woman. In an attempt to achieve closeness with someone, they may choose children, because they feel less likely to be rejected. The sexual element may be linked with the idea of dominance of their partner, which they are unable to achieve in an adult relationship. Sexual activity is mainly confined to genital touching, usually of the child, or in some cases there may be mutual activity or masturbation by the child.

Publicity about paedophilia arises from time to time, when the activities of the Paedophile Information Exchange come to light – perhaps because of a court case, or because changes in the law are sought in order to remove sexual activities with consenting children from the criminal law. Unfortunately, if a paedophile is prosecuted, the trauma to the child may be greater than if a criminal charge is not brought. It is difficult to assess the effect of sexual encounters on children. In Kinsey's survey, 24 per cent of women reported pre-pubertal sexual experiences; he did not ask the same question of men.

It is often suggested that children welcome such approaches, and in some cases this is undoubtedly so, particularly if the child has had little warmth and closeness in his family relationships. A sexual relationship is a means of feeling loved, noticed, of being special, particularly if, as in most cases, violence is not used. Nevertheless, sexual activities with children introduce them to behaviour which is not appropriate for their stage of development, and which may affect their ability to make adult relationships in the future, and as such should not be condoned. It is behaviour which is inappropriate in an adult/child relationship which is one of unequals, in a similar way to the inappropriateness of sexual behaviour between nurse and patient or counsellor and client.

The paedophile, seeking help needs understanding, and an attempt should be made to increase the satisfaction in other areas of his life.

Incest

This is legally defined as sexual intercourse between father/

daughter, mother/son, grandfather/granddaughter, brother/sister. By far the most commonly brought to light is that between father and daughter, 72 per cent in 1973, followed by brother and sister, 24 per cent (Walmsley and White, 1979). However, these figures are for those convicted, and may bear little relationship to incidents occurring.

The age of the child when the offence takes place is most commonly between 13 and 15 years (45.7 per cent), followed by 10 to 12 years (19.4 per cent) and 16 to 17 years (12.4 per cent) (Walmsley and White, 1979). However, although from the same source the figures for under 5 years are nil and 5 to 9 years 7.8 per cent, it is quite possible that incidents happen with younger children where either they do not recognise the incident as anything that should not happen, or that they are unable to tell anyone about it.

Certainly, in my practice I have come across many cases where women have described regular incidents of sexual intercourse with their fathers, at ages of 3 to 8 years, none of which was reported, or even discussed, until they presented to me with sexual problems.

Unfortunately, the conviction of a father, particularly if he is sent away to prison, will compound the guilt that the daughter experiences. In addition to this, the mother, who may well have condoned the relationship, may be very bitter and angry about her husband being sent away and its economic consequences, and may react strongly against the girl.

Incest may produce very conflicting emotions. The girl may be torn between feelings of intense love and closeness for her father, and feelings of betrayal, hate and guilt. This closeness with her father is likely to prevent her from separating from him, and making an adult sexual relationship.

Help is needed so that the girl is able to acknowledge these feelings and to re-establish the links with her mother, who she may need to be able to forgive for allowing the incest to happen.

Rape

In the vast majority of cases, this is sexual assault of women by men, either singly or in groups. However, cases have been described by Sarrel and Masters (1982) where men were raped by women, the anxiety of the situation producing a reflex erection thus allowing them to be mounted.

Rape, which may include other sexual acts such as forced fellatio, is nearly always accompanied by violence (approximately 80 per cent: Bancroft, 1983) and there is controversy over which is the prime motivation – sex or aggression. However, it may not be as simple as that, as Bancroft (1983) suggests a reinforcing link between the two – with the violence leading to a sexual arousal, which reinforces the idea of rape.

It is commonly suggested that the victim knew the rapist, and even that she encouraged the attack. This often adds to the trauma of the victim. She may also experience feelings of guilt that she must have done something to provoke the attack; that she is bad; and may, if she experienced sexual arousal during the attack, see herself as dirty and soiled for ever, and feel acute anxiety whenever she experiences sexual arousal in the future.

Another factor which may add to her guilt feelings is whether or not she resisted the rapist. Women who put up a fight may be treated with more understanding by the police, family and friends. However, women may feel that being raped is preferable to being killed, particularly if faced with a knife or other threats of violence. They are then likely to wonder afterwards 'Could I really have done anything to prevent it?' – particularly if the police suggest that she was really consenting as there were no signs of a struggle.

Legal Rape

One of the particularly difficult aspects of rape, from the legal point of view, is that of the rape of a wife by her husband. The law does not recognise this as marriage carries with it, in law, an automatic consent to intercourse – out of which a woman is unable to opt. However, the Criminal Law Revision Committee has agreed by a majority that the law should be changed. How this will work in practice remains to be seen.

Suggested Further Reading for Part IV

Bancroft, John, *Human Sexuality and its Problems* (Churchill Livingstone, Edinburgh, 1983).

Belliveau, E. and Richter, L., *Understanding Human Sexual Inadequacy* (Hodder and Stoughton, London, 1971).

Forward, S. and Buck. C., *Betrayal of Innocence: Incest and its Devastations* (Penguin, Harmondsworth, 1978).

Kaplan, H.S., *The New Sex Therapy* (Bailliere Tindall, London, 1974).

Tunnadine, P., *Contraception and Sexual Life* (Institute of Psychosexual Medicine, 1970).

PART V

REFERRAL

The previous parts of the book dealt with the communication and counselling skills that the nurse needs before being able to help patients with sexual problems, and the areas of knowledge concerning the development of sexuality, adult sexuality and the causes of sexual problems. Armed with these skills and knowledge, the nurse should feel more able to help patients who have sexual problems.

However, the difficulty for many nurses lies in knowing which patients they are competent to help on their own, how far to go, and at what point they should refer and to whom.

With her knowledge of how the body works and the likely causes of sexual problems, the nurse should be able to form some idea of where the cause of the problem lies – in physical, individual, relationship, educational or situational areas. Some of these areas she will be competent to deal with, others will almost certainly need referral.

Education

With an understanding of normal sexual functioning, the nurse should be competent to deal with problems arising from lack of education in the patient (or couple, it she has an opportunity to talk to both partners). The use of diagrams, models of the reproductive organs, or self-examination by the patient using a mirror, may be helpful. Books, such as *The Book of Love* by David Delvin may be recommended, or others, more specific to the problem.

Situation

As far as situational causes are concerned, often an explanation of how circumstances have an effect on sexual functioning is sufficient to defuse the problem.

However, in many cases, it has to be accepted that nothing can be done to change the situation, even by an experienced counsellor. Where the nurse *can* be of help, is in listening to the problem, giving any relevant information and creating a relationship in which the patient feels that at least someone cares. Nurses usually under-estimate how much they can do in this way, and feel that they have failed if they are unable to offer a solution to the problem.

The remaining causes of sexual problems are more likely to need referral, but before discussing referral agencies, questions surrounding referral need to be considered.

Perhaps the first question to consider is whether or not the patient wishes to be referred. It can be frustrating for the nurse who has taken time to talk with a patient about his problem, and feels that she can offer help by a referral, only to have her offer flatly refused. However, a patient goes through many stages before he is ready for referral. Often the preliminary stages involve talking to a friend, or to his partner; another stage may be mentioning the problem in a casual way at the family planning clinic, to his general practitioner, or when the health visitor or midwife calls. At this stage, there is often no thought of being referred, the patient may just want to off-load some of the tensions surrounding the problem, or want to feel that there is someone to whom he can go if he does decide on referral later. Indeed, the problem may not be as great as the difficulties he feels might be caused by its resolution.

I firmly believe that a patient becomes 'ripe' for referral, and only then will constructive work be able to be done. If, by chance, a patient who has visited his general practitioner and has casually mentioned his sexual problem, is seen by a general practitioner who is keen on referral, the patient may find himself in front of me – looking rather bemused – wondering what on earth he is doing there. Frequently, patients in these circumstances do not accept the appointment offered, or fail to turn up.

Consequently, if the nurse offers the patient the possibility of referral, she need not feel rejected if the offer is not taken up – the offer may be followed up weeks, months or even years later, and so she should make it clear that the patient is free to discuss the matter again if he wishes.

Informal Referral

If the patient has agreed that the nurse may bring someone else in to discuss his problem with him, it may be that an informal referral is the most appropriate. This is likely to be to someone working in the same ward, department, primary health care team or family planning clinic. The person may be another nurse, a doctor or a social worker who is known and accepted by those working together as a team as someone who has greater expertise in the subject. It is unlikely that a letter would be written requesting referral, and reporting back to the referrer is likely to be verbal.

It may be that someone in the area with the specialist knowledge is prepared to discuss problems with the nurse informally, over the telephone or in person, in which case it may be possible for the nurse to continue to see the patient, offering further help after discussion with the specialist source.

Formal Referral

If there is no one to whom an informal approach may be made, then a formal referral is required. The doctor responsible for the medical care of the patient should be consulted, with the patient's permission. This may be a doctor in the clinic, the consultant on the ward, or the general practitioner in the case of health visitors or other community staff.

It is usual for the doctor to make the referral. However, if a nurse has a continuing involvement with the patient, provided that the doctor mentions the nurse in the referral letter, the nurse may well be kept informed about the patient's progress.

Occasionally a patient does not want his general practitioner to know about his referral for advice. In these cases, the nurse should be aware of those in her geographical area who do not insist on referral by a doctor, or who are prepared to take self-referred patients.

Problems of Referral

Occasionally, if the relationship between the nurse and the patient has been over a considerable period of time, then the referral may not be seen in a positive way, but rather as a threat. The need to refer may be seen by the nurse as a sign of failure. She may well feel that she ought to have been able to cope with all the patient's problems. The request for referral by the patient may be felt by the nurse as a rejection of her. Both these examples suggest that the nurse has become too emotionally involved with the patient and needs to stand back and be objective. On the other hand, the patient may see the suggestion of referral by the nurse as a rejection of him, he may feel that she is passing him on because she is tired of him or cannot cope.

The skill of the nurse in referral is to be able to offer referral in such a way that the patient sees it as a positive offer, rather than one of off-loading him – of gaining further expert help, rather than losing someone who is involved in his care. It may be helpful to suggest that the patient returns later to tell the nurse how he got on.

Referral Agencies

It is essential that the nurse is aware of the particular agencies in her area as the facilities vary from one place to another. As well as having knowledge of the agencies, the nurse should know a little about each and about their systems of referral. For example, The Marriage Guidance Council prefers clients to make their own appointments rather than being 'sent'.

The more information that the nurse is able to give the patient about the agency, and preferably about the person to whom he will be referred, the more likely it is that the patient will keep the appointment, and when he does, will need to spend less time testing out the agency to see what is offered. I regularly see patients who believe, erroneously, that they have been sent for surrogate therapy, or that they will be asked to perform, sexually, in front of me.

United Kingdom

The British Association for Counselling has produced a booklet *A Directory of Agencies offering Therapy, Counselling, and Support for Psychosexual Problems*. In the excellent introduction, Elphis Christopher lists the types of therapy currently available.

It may be that some agencies offer mainly one type of therapy, whereas others choose the type of therapy appropriate for the individual patient or for a particular problem. This latter approach is useful as sexual problems may have more than one cause (Christopher, 1983).

Medical Referral. An important factor in referring a patient who has a sexual problem which appears to have a physical cause, is that the doctor to whom the patient is to be referred should have an understanding of sexual problems. This is because some of the investigations which may be required are not part of the routine medical examination. A doctor working in a family planning clinic may be the most appropriate person to reassure a woman that she is 'normal'.

As with all types of referral, facilities for medical referral will differ from place to place. However, consultants from the specialities of gynaecology, urology, neurology, or psychiatry (if she has an interest in the physical aspect) are the most likely to be helpful to patients whose sexual problems appear to have a physical cause.

Psychiatric Departments. Unless she has a particular interest in sexual problems, referral to a psychiatrist is unlikely to be helpful to the patient presenting with sexual problems, unless the patient is mentally ill, or suffering from depression.

If the psychiatrist is also a psychoanalyst, then the type of therapy given is likely to place emphasis on ths difficulties the patient has had in his personal and sexual development. If that is seen by the nurse as the main area of concern, then this may be an appropriate referral for the patient.

Psychology Departments. In some localities, referral to a psychologist must be made through the psychiatric department: in others, direct referral may be made.

Some psychologists are trained in psychotherapeutic methods, which involve the person working out his problem for himself, with the help of the therapist. Again this may be appropriate for those patients with problems of individual development.

Alternatively, psychologists may take a behavioural approach, for example, teaching control of anxiety through desensitisation and relaxation techniques. This approach may be particularly useful for patients with sexual problems in which anxiety plays a large part.

Groups may be run dealing with training in assertiveness, communication and social skills. A patient whose sexual problem is largely the result of difficulty in making relationships may be helped by joining one of these groups.

Sexual Dysfunction Clinics. Some health authorities have special clinics, some of them connected with the psychiatric department, for treating sexual problems. These clinics may be staffed by a multidisciplinary team of psychiatrists, psychologists, nurses and social workers, who may work singly or in pairs as co-therapists. They may use a variety of approaches, combining counselling skills and behavioural techniqes, with the approach being modified to suit the particular patient or problem. Individuals or couples may be seen.

Psychosexual Clinics. These are often connected with family planning clinics, as part of the free health authority service, and are often staffed by doctors who are members of the Institute of Psychosexual Medicine, trained in the Balint approach, in which the interaction between the doctor and patient is focused upon (Balint, 1957).

One of their particular areas of expertise is that of treating women with sexual problems, particularly painful intercourse, vaginismus and non-consummation (Christopher, 1983). Doctors trained in this way are particularly well situated in family planning clinics to pick up and treat sexual dysfunction presented as problems of contraception, or fertility, and may use the genital examination as a therapeutic tool.

The presenting partner, either male or female, is the one likely to be seen, rather than the couple.

General practitioners, who have also been trained in the Balint approach, may specialise in treating patients with sexual problems.

Marriage Guidance Council. Marriage guidance counsellors see individuals or couples (not necessarily married), who present with difficulties in their relationship or personal life.

Patients who have a sexual problem which appears to be a small part of a problem in the general relationship, may benefit from referral to a marriage counsellor. As previously mentioned, patients should, preferably, make the appointment themselves. There may be a small charge, either for registration or for the counselling sessions, depending on the area.

Marriage Guidance Council Marital Sexual Therapy (MST) Clinics
Some marriage counsellors have been trained in the methods of
Masters and Johnson, a behavioural approach. The counsellors
combine their counselling skills with Masters and Johnson techniques and are thus able to treat a wide variety of problems. Counsellors may work in co-therapy teams, and there may be a charge
made.

Private Therapists. It may be that none of the previously mentioned
agencies is within a particular locality, or that a patient wishes to see
a therapist privately.

It is essential to know something of the qualifications and
approach taken by a particular therapist before referral and
personal recommendation by a respected colleague is preferable.

There are two sources of information available in Britain: the
previously mentioned *Directory of Agencies* (See p. 148) offering
counselling and support for psychosexual problems, and a list of
therapists may be obtained from the Association of Sexual and
Marital Therapists.

United States of America

Most sex therapy in the United States is carried out on a private
basis. Consequently, if a nurse in the USA wishes to refer a patient,
then she could contact one of two organisations, who will supply a
list of therapists, if she does not know personally of someone to
whom she may refer patients.

American Association for Marriage and Family Therapy (AAMFT).
In addition to obtaining a list from their main address in Washington DC, the nurse may consult the yellow pages of the local telephone book, where members will be listed.

*American Association of Sex Educators, Counsellors and Therapists
(AASECT).* Address Washington DC.

USEFUL ADDRESSES

Sexual Problems of the Disabled (SPOD)
286 Camden Road
London
N7 OBJ

Association of Sexual and Marital Therapists (ASMT)
PO Box 62
Sheffield
S10 3TS

British Association for Counselling
37A Sheep Street
Rugby
CV21 3BX

Family Planning Information Service
27–35 Mortimer Street
London
W1N 7RJ

Institute of Psychosexual Medicine
111 Harley Street
London
W1N 1DG

National Marriage Guidance Council (NMGC)
Little Church Street
Rugby
CV21 3AP

BIBLIOGRAPHY

Anderson, N.H. (1974) '*Cognitive* Algebra: *Integration Theory Applied to Social Attribution*'. In Berkowitz, L. (ed.), *Advances in Experimental Social Psychology*, Vol. 7 (New York, Academic Press).

Argyle, M. (1972) *The Psychology of Interpersonal Behaviour* (Penguin).

Balint, M. (1957) *The Doctor, His Patient and the Illness* (London, Pitman Medical).

Bancroft, J. (1983) *Human Sexuality and its Problems* (Churchill Livingstone).

Barrett, J.C. and Marshal, J. (1969) 'The Risk of Conception on Different Days of the Menstrual Cycle'. *Population Studies*, 23, 455–61.

Begley, D.J., Firth, J.A., and Hoult, J.R.S. (1980) *Human Reproduction and Developmental Biology* (Macmillan).

Belliveau, E. and Richter, L. (1971) *Understanding Human Sexual Inadequacy* (London, Hodder).

Biestek, F.D. (1967) *The Casework Relationship* (Allen and Unwin).

Bostock, Y. and Leather, D. (1982) 'The Role of Mass Media Advertising Campaigns in Influencing Attitudes towards Contraception in 16–20 Year Olds', *British Journal of Family Planning*, Vol. 8, 59–63.

Brewer, C. (1977) 'Incidence of Post Abortion Psychosis – A Prospective Survey'. *British Medical Journal*, Vol. 1, 476–7.

Chilman, C.S. (1978) *Adolescent Sexuality in a Changing American Society; Social and Psychological Perspectives* (Washington DC, US Department of Health Education and Welfare).

——(1979) 'Teenage Pregnancy: A Research Review'. *Social Work*, Vol. 24, 492–7.

Christopher, E. (1983) Introduction to *Directory of Agencies Offering Counselling and Support for Psychosexual Problems* (British Association for Counselling).

Crisp, A.H. (1980) *Anorexia Nervosa* (Academic Press).

Dallas, D.M. (1972) *Sex Education in School and Society* (National Foundation for Education Research in England and Wales).

Delvin, D. (1974) *The Book of Love* (New English Library).

Ekman, P. (1971) 'Universal and Cultural Differences in Facial Expressions of Emotion'. In Cole, J.K. (ed.), *Nebraska Symposium on Motivation*.

English, O.S. and Pearson, G.H.J. (1965) *Emotional Problems of Living* (Allen and Unwin).

Erikson, E.H. (1963) *Childhood and Society* (New York, W.W. Norton and Co.).

Forward, S. and Buck, C. (1978) *Betrayal of Innocence: Incest and its Devastations*, (Penguin).

French, P. (1983) *Social Skills for Nursing Practice* (London, Croom Helm).

Gagnon, J. and Simon, W. (1973) *Sexual Conduct: The Social Sources of Human Sexuality* (Chicago, Aldine).

George, L. and Weiller, S. (1981) 'Sexuality in Middle and Late Life'. *Archives of General Psychiatry*, Vol. 38, 919–23.

Gittleson, N.L., Eacott, S.E. and Mehta, B.M. (1978) 'Victims of Indecent Exposure'. *British Journal of Psychiatry*, Vol. 132, 61–6.

Glover, J. (1983) 'Sexual Aspects of Parenthood'. *Nursing*, Vol. 2, No. 19, 554–5.

153

Goodwin, R.C. (1969) 'Orgasm and Premature Labour'. *Lancet*, Vol. 2, 646.

Greenacre, P. (1979) 'Fetishism'. In Rosen, I. (ed.), *Sexual Deviations* (Oxford University Press).

Greengross, W. (1976) *Entitled to Love* (National Marriage Guidance Council).

Hamachek, D.E. (1973) 'Development and Dynamics of the Adolescent Self'. In Adams J.F. (ed.), *Understanding Adolescence* (Boston, Allyn and Bacon).

Harlow, H.F. (1959) 'Love in Infant Monkeys', *Scientific American*, June, 68–74.

——(1973) *Learning to Love* (San Francisco, Albion).

Hawkins, D.F. (ed.), (1983) *Drugs and Pregnancy* (Churchill Livingstone).

Hemmings. J., Menzies, M.P., Proops, M. and Fawdry, K. (1971) *Sex Education of School Children* (Royal Society of Health).

Higgins, G.E. (1979) 'Sexual Response in Spinal Cord Injured Adults'. *Archives of Sexual Behaviour*, Vol. 8, 173–96.

Hildegard, E.R., Atkinson, R.C. and Atkinson, R.L. (1979) *Introduction to Psychology* (Harcourt Brace Jovanovich).

Hockey, L. (1976) *Women in Nursing* (Hodder and Stoughton).

Kahn, J.H. (1971) *Human Growth and Development of Personality* (Pergamon Press).

Kalodny, R.C., Masters, W.H. and Johnson, V.E. (1979) *Textbook of Sexual Medicine* (Boston, Little, Brown and Co.).

Kaplan, H.S. (1974) *The New Sex Therapy* (London, Balliere Tindall).

——(1979) *Disorders of Sexual Desire* (Balliere Tindall).

Kinsey, A.G., Pomeroy, W.B., and Martin, C.F. (1948) *Sexual Behaviour in the Human Male* (Philadelphia, Saunders).

Lowe, G.R. (1972) *The Growth of Personality* (Pelican).

Masters, W.H. and Johnson, V.E. (1966) *Human Sexual Response* (Boston, Little, Brown and Co.).

——(1970) *Human Sexual Inadequacy* (London, Churchill).

Munro, M.S. (1979) *Counselling – A Skills Approach* (Methuen Publications New Zealand).

Nurse, G. (1975) *Counselling and the Nurse* (Aylesbury, H.M. and M. Publishers).

Philips, J.C., Jnr. (1969) *The Origins of Intellect – Piaget's Theory* (San Francisco, W.H. Freeman).

Renvoise, J. (1982) *Incest: A Family Pattern* (Penguin).

Rogers, C. (1965) *Client Centred Therapy* (Constable).

Rooth, F.G. (1972) 'Changes in Conviction Rate for Indecent Exposure', *British Journal of Psychiatry*, Vol. 121, 89–94.

Sarrel, P. and Masters, W.H. (1982) 'Sexual Molestation of Men by Women'. *Archives of Sexual Behaviour*, Vol. 11, 2.

Specht, R. and Craig, C.J. (1982) *Human Development* (Prentice Hall)

Stewart, W. (1979) *The Sexual Side of Handicap* (Cambridge, Woodhead Falkner).

Tanner, J.M. (1971) *Sequence, Tempo and Individual Development of Boys and Girls Aged Twelve to Sixteen* (Daedalus).

Thomas, A., Chess, S. and Birch, H.G. (1970) 'The Origin of Personality'. *Scientific American*, Vol. 223, 2, 102–9.

Tietze, C. (1960) 'Probability of Pregnancy Resulting from a Single Unprotected Coitus', *Fertility and Sterility*, Vol. 2, 485–8.

Tietze, C. *et al.* (1979) 'USA Data'. *International Journal of Gynaecology and Obstetrics*, Vol. 16, 456.

Tunnadine, P. (1970) *Contraception and Sexual Life* (Institute of Psychosexual Medicine).

Wagner, G. and Green, R. (1981) *Impotence* (New York, Plenum Press).

Walmsley, R. and White, K. (1979) 'Sexual Offences, Consent and Sentencing', *Home Office Research Study No. 54* (London, HMSO).

Wilson, G.T. and Lawson, D.M. (1976) 'Expectancies, Alcohol and Sexual Arousal in Male Social Drinkers'. *Journal of Abnormal Psychology*, Vol. 85, 587–94.

Zelnik, M. and Kanther, J. (1977) 'Sexual and Contraceptive Experiences of Young Women in the United States 1971–1976'. *Family Planning Perspectives* (March – April).

Zilbergeld, B. (1978) *Men and Sex* (Fontana).

INDEX

parasympathetic nervous system 74,
    76
parents
    and adolescents 54, 56
    and handicapped children 106–7
    and Oedipal situation 42–3
    and sex education 59–60
    influence on sexual development 40,
        52, 111
    of stillborn baby 99
partner
    belittling 128
    over-demanding 128
    unresponsive 128
patient
    bodyspace 14
    hand on the door 14, 25
    'special pearl' 20
    whole person 1
peer group 48, 53–6, 61, 97
pelvic inflammatory disease 121
pelvis 74, 78
penetration
    fear of 85
penis 71–4, 79, 118, 132–3
    and self esteem 126, 128
    envy 41, 124
    glans 71
    in puberty 51–3
    prepuce 71
perception 9–11, 29, 50, 61
perineum 68, 74
periods 47, 103
    see also menstruation
peripheral neuropathy 119, 123
personality 123, 125–6, 137
petting 85, 112
Peyronies Disease 121
phimosis 121
physical problems 2, 18, 117–23
physically handicapped 106–7
Piaget, J. 34
pill 57, 111
    see also combined pill
pituitary 50
plateau 79, 80
playleader 63
posterior fornix 69–70
post-natal 95–6
pre-eclampsia 93
pregnancy 92–6
    and adolescents 55, 58
    and sex eduation 60–1
    chance of 92
    fears of 18, 94, 111, 135

intercourse in 93, 96
    unwanted 96
premature ejaculation 38, 88, 115,
    116, 134
premature labour 93
presenting problem 19, 20
priapism 121
privacy 4, 94, 107
    for counselling 21, 25
    for sexual relationships 83–4, 134
progesterone 51, 122
prolactin 76, 92, 95, 122
prostaglandins 93
prostate 51, 73
prostatectomy 79, 115, 121
psychiatric department 149, 150
    disorders 122
    hospitals 4
    patients 4
psychiatrist 149–50
psychoanalyst 149
psychologists 149–50
psychosexual clinic 150
psychotrophic drugs 122
    see also tranquilisers
puberty 40, 50–3, 71
public health nurse 3
pudenal nerve 74
puerpium 3

questioning 27

rape 45, 111–12, 143–4
    legal 144
reassurance 27, 39
record keeping 30–1
rectum 68
referral 23, 32
    agencies 148–51
    assessment for 146
    formal 147
    informal 147
    medical 149
    problems with 147
reflect 28, 31
reflex action 37
    arc 74
refractory period 80, 105, 115, 117
regional differences 9
regression 34, 44
relationships
    affect of childhood development on
        36, 38, 123
    in adolescence 55
    in handicap 107

COL. & MRS. S. C. CRAXFORD
12 ETHELBERT DRIVE
CHARLTON NEAR ANDOVER
HANTS. SP10 4ET
TEL. ANDOVER (0264) 50220